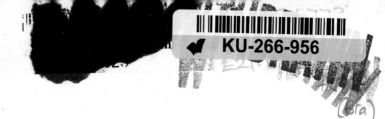
HEALTH
PROMOTION
AT THE
COMMUNITY
LEVEL
2

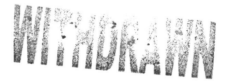
1

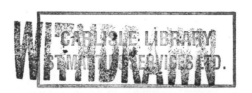

Go in search of people.
Begin with what they know.
Build on what they have.

—Old Chinese proverb

NEIL BRACHT

editor

HEALTH PROMOTION AT THE COMMUNITY LEVEL

2

New Advances

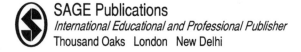

SAGE Publications
International Educational and Professional Publisher
Thousand Oaks London New Delhi

For information:

 SAGE Publications, Inc.
2455 Teller Road
Thousand Oaks, California 91320
E-mail: order@sagepub.com

SAGE Publications Ltd.
6 Bonhill Street
London EC2A 4PU
United Kingdom

SAGE Publications India Pvt. Ltd.
M-32 Market
Greater Kailash I
New Delhi 110 048 India

Printed in the United States of America

Library of Congress Cataloging-in-Publication Data

Main entry under title:

Health promotion at the community level: New advances /
    edited by Neil Bracht.—2nd ed.
        p. cm.
    Includes bibliographical references and index.
    ISBN 0-7619-1844-2 (cloth: acid-free paper)
    ISBN 0-7619-1304-1 (pbk.: acid-free paper)
    1. Health promotion. 2. Community health services—
Citizen participation. I. Bracht, Neil F.
    RA427.8 .H494 1998
    362.1'0425—dc21   98-40267

    00   01   02   03   10   9   8   7   6   5   4   3

Acquiring Editor:	Jim Nageotte
Editorial Assistant:	Heidi Van Middlesworth
Production Editor:	Diana E. Axelsen
Editorial Assistant:	Nevair Kabakian
Typesetter/Designer:	Marion Warren
Indexer:	Virgil Diodato
Cover Designer:	Candice Harman

Contents

PART II
Cross-National Experiences: Issues in Developing and Sustaining Community Health Programs

Foreword

A modern, international movement termed _health promotion_ has emerged out of the historical need for a fundamental change in strategy to achieve and maintain health. During the initial era of public health, concern about communicable diseases appropriately dominated thinking. That led to the "cleanup" campaigns of the 19th century and, later, to the discovery of microbiologic agents of disease and the development of means for their control. Breaking the chain of infection became the focus of attention, later supplemented by strengthening people's resistance: sewage disposal, water treatment, pasteurization of milk, food protection, and avoidance of crowding. These actions, directed at preventing the spread of infectious agents and bolstered by immunizations against specific diseases, proved remarkably effective against the major health problems of the day.

But another day has brought new health problems, a new system responsible for their origin, and a new set of requirements for their control. The current major problems, mainly the chronic diseases of middle and later life, arise out of conditions to which people are exposed when they enter modern industrialized life and out of their response to those conditions: plenty of calories, especially in the form of fats; lessened demands for physical exertion and heightened demands on the psyche; easy access to tobacco and excessive amounts of alcohol; and motor vehicle transport. Interaction of people with that new milieu constitutes the system that has generated present-day epidemics such as cardiovascular disease, cancer, chronic respiratory disease, cirrhosis, trauma, and diabetes.

Again, scientific progress has disclosed enough about the nature of the current human-environment-disease system for the social organization of health advance. Breaking the chain of infection and building human resistance to it will no longer suffice. It has become necessary (a) to establish health-protective social policies concerning those aspects of life in industrialized societies that seriously jeopardize health and (b) to help people cope with such conditions of life so long as they exist.

In former times, social action against principal health problems consisted largely of erecting physical barriers to the transmission of disease agents and providing immunizations. It also included attention to the medical needs of mothers and children. Education of people concerning personal hygiene, such as hand washing and sputum control, and other aspects of health played some role. The situation, however, induced action mainly toward environmental protection.

Now recognition has grown that people's behavior in their present milieu and the conditions of life that influence behavior, rather than direct physical exposure to biological disease agents, constitute the major health issue. The social environment—especially access and encouragement to indulge in tobacco, excessive alcohol, and calories and too little physical exercise—has become more significant for health nowadays than physical environmental hazards. That is the reason for the profound shift in health strategy.

Progress in the new situation has been under way for some time. Exercise is trendy in some circles and seat belt use is up, but not all signs are favorable. Obesity continues at a high level and even appears to be increasing. Some segments of the population lag seriously in overcoming behavior that is adverse to health. For example, people with low educational levels continue to smoke cigarettes, and their children also become addicted to nicotine. Teen smoking is once again on the increase.

Corresponding to the generally positive behavior changes, along with some medical advances, coronary heart disease mortality has fallen sharply, and the lung cancer epidemic has reached its peak among men. People have started learning, as individuals, to cope with the conditions of life that induce these and other principal diseases. More important for the long term, they have initiated social changes to create a more healthful milieu in which to live. Thus television advertising of cigarettes has been banned in the United States, and smoking is prohibited in many places. Some states have increased taxes on tobacco products as a measure against their use. Progress internationally is well documented in Part II of this revised edition.

Health promotion is thus advancing worldwide. This book is designed to guide professionals in both the health and community organization fields as well as interested citizens in their actions to improve community health. The book's significance lies in its potential to accelerate favorable trends and commence additional ones. A far cry from earlier efforts aimed directly at influencing individuals to adopt healthier patterns, the emphasis here is on the community. As editor, Neil Bracht has sought deliberately to bring together what has been learned in recent years about community organization processes and community intervention strategies and demonstrate the applicability of this knowledge to the health field.

In so doing, he gives recognition to the fact that although individuals act in ways that affect health, the community largely determines individuals' actions. Hence, the focus here is on communitywide health promotion. Norms are established at the community level and transmitted to individuals as strong guidance. Realizing that relationship and building health promotion strategy clearly geared to it should help overcome the lingering resistance to health promotion as "blaming the victim." Social action is needed for health promotion. It must be directed principally at the social situations that influence people's health-related behavior rather than at the physical environment that impinges on health without the intermediary of individual behavior. The task of perfecting the physical environment for health is by no means complete, but the new health environment now requires greater attention to such social forces as the extensive advertising of alcohol, widespread portrayal of alcohol use in films and television as "the thing to do," inadequate constraint of driving while intoxicated, and low taxes on alcoholic beverages. These circumstances exert a profound effect on health.

This volume offers substantial help to those interested in the community approach to health promotion. It reflects the considerable knowledge gained in the past 10 years. It outlines principles and practical advice concerning important aspects of organizing for communitywide health promotion, such as how to use local media while operating within budget constraints, patterns of academic-community relationships, participation of local health professionals, implications of worksite health promotion experience for other organized groups, involving people in evaluation, and institutionalization of efforts initiated from outside the community. These and other issues addressed here immediately confront those who undertake health promotion in the community. Programs in underserved communities are insightfully described to indicate the special problems in those segments of the population.

This new edition makes a valuable contribution to the field.

—LESTER BRESLOW, M.D., M.P.H.
Center for Health Promotion
UCLA School of Public Health

Acknowledgments

Community health promotion has advanced greatly over the past two decades and is energetically approaching a "third generation" of research and development. The advances reported in this second edition owe much to the pioneering work of the "first generation" of community health promoters: those researchers, funding agencies, and community groups responsible for earlier intervention trials and projects. The researchers, many of whom made contributions to the first edition of this book, provided an important foundation for the growth and dissemination of the health promotion movement seen today. The lessons of these earlier studies, when coupled with the current insights of more comprehensive community health and social initiatives, provide for a growing science of community behavioral and environmental risk reduction. Equally important is our understanding of the key indicators of successful community participation that have evolved from these more recent experiences.

The results of community intervention trials and studies are mixed, and they present challenges to the funding and design of new initiatives. Although puzzling, these challenges have not deterred the authors of this volume in their attempts to improve global health, equity, and community development. These contributors share a positive view of advances both made and yet to be clarified. I deeply appreciate their sustained interest in, and contributions to, this publication "partnership."

The global nature of the health promotion movement offers a far richer base for understanding the common strategies and principles of community health promotion. Part II of this second edition is almost entirely a report on selected international studies and developments. I am indebted to my former Minnesota colleague, Dr. Maurice Mittelmark, for encouraging a "course correction" away from the mostly North American approach of the first edition. No one scientific approach or model can embrace the richness of cross-national experimentation and development one now observes. Dr. Mittelmark, now of the University of Bergen, adeptly captures this diversity in the lead chapter for this book. He reviews the work, findings, and approaches of many studies worldwide. Both Dr. Mittelmark's and my own association with the World Health Organization's health promotion and Healthy Cities movements have enriched our understanding of broader health and social development opportunities. Dr. Mittelmark was a major editorial adviser for Part II of this book, and I am most appreciative of his overall commitment to the work of the second edition.

I was particularly fortunate to have had the opportunity to personally observe the work of recent studies in Canada focused on the dissemination process of health intervention strategies. Several provinces in collaboration with "Health Canada" are undertaking important investigations of successful dissemination approaches. A special thanks to volunteers and colleagues on Prince Edward Island for sharing their promising approach to community empowerment and sustainability.

Dr. Beti Thompson's pioneering contribution, in the first edition, on social change in the community (updated here) is now enlarged with her lead chapter for Part II of the book, which explores strategic planning for durability of health promotion efforts. Among the original authors, she was first to politely suggest that the time for a second edition was overdue. Our ongoing dialogue has been immensely helpful in the development of this "new advances" edition. I am, of course, thankful to Dr. Terry Pahacek, who first suggested that a book such as this would be useful to the field and did much to support the work of the first edition.

Closer to home, I have continued to be the beneficiary of an ongoing association with outstanding colleagues and scholars in the Division of Epidemiology at the University of Minnesota. I especially want to thank Dr. Russell Luepker, Chair of the division, for his long-standing support of my work. His national and international contributions to the science of community health promotion and epidemiology are well known. His earlier first edition contribution (with Dr. Lennart Rastam) on physician involvement in community studies has led to a rich and widely available literature on the critical nature of physician roles in health promotion. Dr. John Finnegan has been a close working research colleague who has made unique contributions to understanding the ties between media campaigns and the community organization components of community trials. His insights, including new web page protocols for community implementation, have been extremely useful to me and research colleagues elsewhere. To many other faculty in "Epi" I express my thanks for being able to share so directly in the exceptional quality of your research, including innovative training programs for future community health professionals.

Disseminating the theory and science of community health promotion has been a special contribution of the many staff members and professionals in the Minnesota Department of Health. I appreciate the numerous opportunities for collaboration with the department, and I especially thank Lee Kingsbury, senior planner, who is pioneering new linkages between managed care and public health (see Chapter 12). The department's partnerships with a wide range of voluntary and public groups have provided expanded field laboratory settings for studying issues of implementation, citizen participation, and empowerment. This has also been true on my visits to many other Public Health Departments, in this country and abroad, where I have observed the unique features and challenges of community partnerships.

Many of the opportunities I have had to observe and learn have come from invitations to consult on a number of long-term studies funded by the National Heart, Lung, and Blood Institute (NHLBI), National Cancer Institute (NCI), and Centers for Disease Control (CDC), among others. Particularly useful in this regard were the Community Intervention Trial for Smoking Cessation (COMMIT) and American Stop Smoking Intervention for Cancer Prevention (ASSIST) projects of NCI and the Rapid Early Action for Coronary Treatment (REACT) project of NHLBI. The scientific and professional staff of the NIH Institutes who have supported my participation in these and related studies are too numerous to mention, but clearly, I owe much to many. This sentiment of appreciation applies equally to staff members of several foundations (e.g., Kaiser, Robert Wood Johnson, and California Wellness) who have made significant investments in the community-based health movement. I have also benefited from my association with the Society of Public Health Education (SOPHE).

It is my hope that those leaders of governmental and private organizations who have invested substantially in community-based health studies will remember that positive outcomes often take longer than anticipated. This has been shown in one of the original community-based studies—the North Karelia Project in Finland. Also, let's not forget that sometimes we learn as much from mixed or negative results as we do from positive ones. Federal and state legislative groups, along with their counterparts in the foundations, need to stay the course in funding important but unfinished research agendas. Future investments in community development for health will help us better determine the "right mix" of actions required to effectively mobilize communities and improve social and health conditions.

As I mentioned in the acknowledgment to the first edition, many insights, both about the science and art of community work, continue to come from the volunteer community groups and leaders I have collaborated with over the years. Equally valuable are the insights and hindsight of the numerous community organizers and project field directors who have given of their time in training and evaluative feedback sessions, sharing their perspectives on what works, what doesn't, and why. The accumulated wisdom of these groups has too rarely been captured in the subject literature. What I have learned from them I have integrated into the content of this book (especially in Chapter 4). As I now devote more of my professional career effort to community health development, consultation, and training over the next few years, I anticipate even more productive exchanges with the above-mentioned groups.

Finally, I wish to thank my wife and family for their support throughout this process.

—NEIL BRACHT
University of Minnesota

Introduction

This book is about ways to improve the health of communities. There is a new urgency to the complex and important work of advancing community health promotion activities and policies. Population groups around the world are experiencing sharp declines in earlier achieved health gains. Life expectancy in Eastern Europe is declining. In Russia, for example, life expectancy in men declined from 64 years in 1989 to 57.2 years in 1996. In Zimbabwe, largely because of deaths from AIDS, life expectancy, now age 61, is projected to be age 49 by the end of this century. The 1998 International AIDS Conference in Geneva labeled AIDS a "runaway epidemic." Africa has 90% of all AIDS deaths in the world, and thousands of children are being left to care for themselves. By the year 2000, the World Health Organization estimates that 16 million women worldwide will be infected with HIV. The social and economic costs of coronary disease continue despite much knowledge of modifiable risk factors. The second International Heart Health Conference in Barcelona (1995) predicted a rise to 20 million cardiovascular deaths by the year 2005, with 13 million of these in developing countries and Eastern Europe.

All of these statistics and trends are troubling enough, but when coupled with the negative health indicators from more industrialized/Western countries, the call for bold new investments in health promotion programs, training, and research becomes more pressing. In the United States, nearly half of the 3 to 5 million migrant and seasonal farmworkers have positive tuberculosis skin tests. Hispanic women of Mexican and Puerto Rican origin are at significantly higher risk of AIDS and cervical cancer than the general U.S. population (Suarez & Siefert, 1998). Latinas are among the youngest and fastest growing minority group in the United States, and they must be a high priority for prevention work, along with other high-risk groups. Substance abuse and cigarette smoking among young people are at unacceptable levels, not to mention increased violence on streets and in schools. Twenty-five percent of 12th graders in U.S. schools smoke regularly. New data show an increase in smoking among African American and Hispanic youth (America's Children, 1998). Revised estimates of the number of overweight or obese Americans are now at 97 million. A recent study (Ebrahim, 1998) found that the prevalence of alcohol use by pregnant women increased from 9.5% to 15.3% from 1992 to 1995. Refugee health and mental health problems continue to be a serious concern in the United States and in other countries as well (Dhooper & Tran, 1998).

What all of these negative indicators of health status have in common is that they are largely amenable to health promotion and/or preventive community action. Communities and their governmental entities can mobilize to successfully reduce social, behavioral, and environmental risks to health. For example, high blood lead levels among U.S. children have decreased signifi-cantly over the past two decades as a result of concerted social action. This book's chapters and case studies point to numerous other successful projects that promote health and prevent unneces-sary illness. Much can be learned from a worldwide sharing of health promotion experience, and each author of this edition lists lessons learned in his or her specific content area. The general strategies and approaches required to successfully confront the deterioration of global health status are well-known. They were succinctly outlined in the first International Health Conference on Health Promotion (Ottawa Charter, 1986) and in subsequent conferences (Adelaide, 1988; Sundsvall, Sweden, 1991; Jakarta, 1997). These include five primary strategies:

- Build healthy public policy.
- Create supportive environments.
- Strengthen community action.
- Develop personal skills.
- Reorient health services.

With these overall strategies and guides as background, the chapters of this volume add the tested science and practice skills content required for effective and accountable community health promotion. The authors demonstrate in considerable detail how health promotion programs are implemented and evaluated and how the lives of citizens and the community they live in can be improved. This is a book about both the art and science of community-based health work, and it will be useful to laypersons and professionals alike. At the heart of any successful community health effort is capacity building and local empowerment. This book also provides tangible suggestions for assisting citizens, governmental agencies, and voluntary health groups to collabo-rate and advocate for healthy community policies. Such policies will be sustained only if the political will and vision remain strong and are periodically reinforced.

The last decade of research and development has considerably advanced the science of what Lester Breslow, in the Foreword, refers to as "a modern, international movement [that] emerged out of the historical need for a fundamental change in strategy to achieve and maintain health." The vitality of future population-based health and social improvements will demand continuing attention to discover what works, what doesn't, and why. Our understanding is improving, and more remains to be learned both nationally and internationally. In this second edition, the contributing authors share their "lessons learned" from diverse health promotion experiences and point out areas requiring further study and/or adjustment in community implementation.

The growth of the movement will be further enhanced through the refinement of community organization processes enabling local citizens and groups to participate fully in actions to promote healthy communities. Green (1990) stated it best in the first edition: "community development puts the control over the determinants of health where it belongs—with the people." Empowerment theory is emphasized in Chapter 4 and is a recurring theme in many chapters and case studies within the book.

One "threat" to community empowerment comes from externally designed research proto-cols that include little, if any, community input. Mittelmark's (1990) earlier chapter contribution on "Balancing the Requirements of Research and the Needs of Communities" has helped to sensitize a generation of health promotion practitioners to the negotiations required in community work. In fact, more participatory evaluation initiatives between researchers and community representatives are now being reported in the literature. This is a welcome advance. Beti Thompson and Carol Winner enlarge this dialectic of community versus research interests (see this edition's Chapter 7, on the durability of health promotion) when they discuss the tension between scientific integrity and broad public health dissemination of partially tested interventions.

As indicated earlier, this revised edition has been expanded to better integrate the international dimension(s) of health promotion. Part II of the book reports on recent health promotion programs and health policy developments from several continents. Although not exhaustive, these selective experiences provide the reader with a broader perspective and richness to the work of health promotion and community involvement. In sum, these new chapters are a potent reminder of the importance of culture, geography, and politics in shaping health and healthy environments.

In the lead chapter to the book, Maurice B. Mittelmark summarizes the wide range of definitions and approaches to health promotion and critically examines the mixed scientific results from numerous large-scale community-based studies. His past research in North America, current work in Europe, and frequent interchange with the World Health Organization uniquely qualify him for this daunting task. Part I of the book provides for the core theory and practice principles of community-based health promotion. It builds on the foundation content that readers found most useful from the first edition; this foundation is now updated and linked with three new case studies that immediately follow the conceptual and theory content of Chapters 2, 3, and 4. Case study authors bring a rich background of experience in both quantitative and qualitative research designs, practical field operations, and proven results in fostering community participation.

In Chapter 2, Beti Thompson and Susan Kinne review past and current theories of social change. A wide range of individual, organizational, community, and environmental change theories are analyzed and synthesized. She discusses the lack of empirical attention paid to studying changes in norms and values and how this is tied to the lack of an integrated theoretical explanation of community change. Suggestions for improved community measures are made. A successful cancer prevention screening project from North Carolina is used to illustrate the use of a theory-driven intervention.

In Chapter 3, models and methods for conducting a comprehensive community needs assessment and resource(s) analysis are presented by Chris Rissel, a colleague from Australia. Again, this builds on the earlier first edition chapter but reflects more of a "community strengths" perspective. A case study (conducted by the research team from the University of Vermont Health Promotion Center) on community capacity building in Florida follows. Themes of empowerment, durability, and accurate needs assessments emanate from this rich case history.

In Chapter 4, the applied process of mobilizing citizens and organizations to empower communities for effective health and social improvement is detailed. This is an updated version of the five-stage community organization model presented in the first edition (Bracht and Kingsbury, Chapter 3) but with an enlarged focus on empowerment theory (Rissel), coalition building, and advocacy. The chapter discusses optional organizational structures in building successful citizen involvement in community and health development. References to a substantial number of other works and community participation experiences are provided. A rural case study using the five-stage community organization model follows the chapter, explicating the principles of community mobilization and intervention.

Most would agree that mass media campaigns can be an important aspect of successful community health intervention projects for social change. Increased experience with message design, marketing, and the phasing of campaign interventions provides new lessons for using local and regional media channels. John R. Finnegan Jr. and his colleague K. Viswanath review these recent innovations, which include more interactive media possibilities. Web site educational programs for professionals and community leaders are also mentioned. The implications for public health practice are changing dramatically, and this chapter provides an essential framework for improving the use of media, especially in reaching low socioeconomic and low literacy groups.

Part I of the book concludes with an updated chapter by Phyllis L. Pirie on the challenges and approaches to evaluating health promotion programs. This readily understood content should be useful to a diverse audience of researchers, professionals, community citizens, and students but especially to those new to health promotion activities. Formative, process, and outcome evaluation measures are highlighted.

As mentioned above, Part II of the book focuses more specifically on international developments. Issues of durability, centralization versus decentralization, infrastructure support, and broad intersectoral approaches are common themes among these varied reports. This section of the book begins with a discussion by Beti Thompson and Carol Winner of the durability of community intervention programs, a topic of increasing cross-national interest. The content on durability is new and brings a much-needed framework for examining this important dimension of local and national health promotion programming. Too many public agencies and nongovernmental organizations ignore this aspect of planning and policy resource development. Though limited, recent evidence as presented in this chapter suggests that when durability planning is integrated into a community-based project or governmental initiative, ongoing actions and policies can continue. Community groups and partnerships often want programs to continue and have the motivation to secure resources for long-term impact. Following descriptions of health promotion programs in Africa (Knut-Inge Klepp and colleagues), Asia (Rhonda Galbally and colleagues), Latin America (Abel Arvizu Whittemore and Janet R. Buelow), and Nordic and related countries of Europe (John G. Maeland and Bo J.A. Haglund), Part II concludes with the discussion of an emerging development in the United States. This development relates to achieving community health goals through collaborations between traditional public health agencies and private medical care groups, especially large managed care systems. Lee Kingsbury provides some early insights into the promise and barriers of such arrangements and lists some of the early lessons learned. These emerging partnerships, which are unique to the entrepreneurial aspects of the American health system, may well have broader applications for public-private interactions elsewhere.

Finally, it should be obvious to all who engage in the work of improving communities that communities, however defined, are undergoing tremendous changes. Individuals and families are buffeted by social, economic, and environmental forces that weaken ties of mutual support. Social disconnectedness increases the opportunities for violence and discrimination. The ravages of war and famine continue to dislocate and alienate large numbers of people worldwide. Inequality of education and income deprive many of their fullest potential. These conditions, as well as the alarming deterioration of health status mentioned at the beginning of this Introduction, must receive critical and sustained attention now. This book can help to foster the work yet to be done to achieve healthy communities and healthy nations.

—NEIL BRACHT
University of Minnesota

PART I

Advances in the Theory and Practice of Community Health Promotion

CHAPTER 1

Health Promotion at the Communitywide Level

Lessons From Diverse Perspectives

MAURICE B. MITTELMARK

This is an account of some of the key lessons that have been learned during the past several decades concerning planning, implementing, and researching health promotion at the communitywide level. The spatial or geopolitical boundaries within which programs take place and the complexity and extent of community action can vary widely. A small group of individuals working on improving safety conditions in their immediate neighborhood is an example of relatively small-scale action. A citywide, multisector coalition working on injury prevention operates on a much larger scale. The term communitywide describes large-scale programs that are intended to involve many residents and the institutions of entire villages, towns, or cities.

It is natural that many health promoters have been eager to undertake their work at this level of human organization. Villages, towns, and cities are where people gather, live, work, learn, love, and play. The social and physical environments at the communitywide level have significant influence on the well-being of individuals who live in the community and who, in turn, influence their environment and thus the well-being of others. The many settings of which communities are composed (schools and workplaces, for example) provide multiple opportunities to involve residents of all ages and walks of life in health promotion.

It has also been natural that many health promotion research projects have been conducted at the communitywide level. Communities at this level are highly organized, and local government, businesses, schools, churches, clubs, neighborhood associations, and media can all be engaged on behalf of health promotion. This provides the possibility for intense and sustained intervention.

AUTHOR'S NOTE: The author gratefully acknowledges the assistance of Professors Henry Blackburn, David Jacobs, and Don Nutbeam, whose critical reviews of an earlier version of this chapter were most helpful.

Large towns and cities contain, also, enough people to accommodate a wide range of research approaches, from the epidemiological to the sociological.

It is not surprising, then, that during the past several decades, hundreds of health promotion demonstration or research projects have been conducted at the communitywide level. In searching out key lessons from the experiences of these projects, the reach must be international, as health promotion at the communitywide level has been undertaken in communities all over the globe. The reach must also be selective, to complement the material presented elsewhere in this volume and to respect the limits of space. Accordingly, two main streams of experience provide the foci of this treatment: cardiovascular disease prevention research on the one hand and community development for health promotion on the other. In-depth examination of two very divergent approaches to health promotion, as these are, sharpens critical perspective and illustrates healthy diversity in approaches to health promotion at the communitywide level.

Some of the lessons recounted here are prescriptive. Based on evidence, certain approaches, practices, and strategies seem to be fundamental to successful communitywide health promotion efforts. Some of the lessons remain somewhat speculative, as they are lessons drawn more from what has not happened than from what has happened. Some of the lessons are conditional. One size does not fit all. Not least, some of the lessons are controversial. Health promotion as a field of practice and an arena of research is far from mature enough to hope for consensus on many important issues.

Health Promotion's Diversity

The remarkable range of issues to which community-based health promotion has been applied is illustrated in part by several other chapters in this volume, such as the prevention of HIV/AIDS and injuries, yet this is but a sampling of the possibilities. A reasonably complete listing would have to include, for example, violence reduction among African and Hispanic American youth (Wiist, Jackson, & Jackson, 1996), mosquito larval control in Honduras (Leontsini, Gil, Kendall, & Clark, 1993), mental health promotion in Norway (Sorensen, Boe, Ingebrigtsen, & Sandanger, 1996), prevention of developmental disabilities (Adams & Hollowell, 1992), promotion of breast feeding in Mexico (Rodriguez-Garcia, Aumack, & Ramos, 1990), and asthma management in the U.S. (Fisher et al., 1996).

An even more inclusive review would encompass programs aiming to improve the social, environmental, economic, and political determinants of health. Examples include empowerment, capacity-building, and sustainable development in Latin America (Markides & Garrett, 1996), building local-private partnerships to develop local enterprise zones (Watson, 1995), tourism development, building on natural resources in Indonesia (Long & Wall, 1996), creation of new resources to save rural communities, such as the building of gaming attractions in the American Midwest (Long, 1996), and development of Local Exchange Trading Systems (LETS), in which members exchange goods and services based on locally developed units of exchange instead of national currencies (Thorne, 1996; Williams, 1996).

Despite the obvious heterogeneity of projects such as these, two broad, distinguishing themes are discernible. First, there are many programs that have as their main objective(s) the prevention of specific diseases, illnesses, and symptoms, and/or the promotion of specific health outcomes. Such health promotion programs are frequently a part of formal research projects. They are often managed by academics who work in partnership with specific communities selected by the researchers. They employ hypothesis-testing research methods to assess a program's ability to achieve significant improvements in the specific health issue that is the program focus. Such programs are often underwritten by external (to the community) research and demonstration grants in combination with contributions from the participating communities. The most important of such contributions is the time that citizens contribute as volunteers.

Examples of this type are to be found among the many community-based research and demonstration programs for the prevention of the cardiovascular diseases, diabetes, cancers, and their risk factors (Carrageta, Negrao, & de-Padua, 1994; Hancock et al., 1996; Heath, Wilson, Smith, & Leonard, 1991; Herbert, 1996; Holm et al., 1989; Kreuter, 1992; O'Neill, Pederson, & Rootman, 1994; Puska, 1988; Shea & Basch, 1990).

Disease Prevention

Of all the objectives to which communitywide health promotion has been directed, the prevention of cardiovascular diseases (CVD) has had the highest priority worldwide, by a very wide margin. This has been a natural and reasoned response to epidemiological evidence that the largest burden of morbidity and mortality is attributable in most developed societies to the cardiovascular diseases (Epstein, 1992; Marmot, 1992). Further, these diseases are influenced to a degree by lifestyle factors that seem readily modifiable through a combination of medical therapy and behavior change techniques (Blackburn, 1992; Rose, 1992).

Four cardiovascular disease prevention research projects in particular have had enormous impact on the way health promotion at the community level is conducted. These projects, from Finland (Puska, 1988), California (Farquhar, 1978), Rhode Island (Lasater et al., 1984), and Minnesota (Blackburn et al., 1984) are the main exemplars from which lessons are drawn about disease prevention practice and research at the communitywide level. There are, of course, other important examples of community-based cardiovascular disease prevention research initiatives, such as the Canadian Heart Health Initiative (Stachenko, 1996) and the German Cardiovascular Prevention Study (Hoffmeister et al., 1996), to mention but two prominent programs. However, the intention here is to examine a limited number of exemplars very closely, and the Finnish and American studies selected are sufficiently similar in project design and implementation to permit the necessary contrasts and comparisons.

Community Development

In the other program type, the main objective is community development for health promotion. These programs focus on building community capacities to mount and manage many different kinds of health promotion programs or to improve the basic foundations for a thriving community, such as equitable access to education and economic security, social connectedness of the citizenry, and public policy that supports agreed-on health objectives. Such programs may have a specific health or human development issue as their raison d'être, such as promoting a healthy social and physical environment in which to raise children. The special challenge of community development is how to recognize, use, and increase the capacities and resources within the community, as opposed to depending on a significant infusion of resources from outside the community. In its ideal form, community development arises from the grass roots of the community itself. In practice, community development for health promotion is often initiated or at least stimulated by community elites or by outsiders.

Community development research is frequently constructed as "participatory action research," an approach in which community members are involved in the research as partners, at every stage of a project (Flynn, Ray, & Rider, 1994; Rains & Ray, 1995; Whyte, 1991). Such research is without a formal hypothesis testing research component, but it does often have evaluation components to monitor activity, studies to document program processes and activities, and research to help improve the effectiveness of action. These are often coordinated by public or private agencies (international, national, regional) that are positioned to serve as consultants and advisors to communities. Usually, communities elect actively to participate, pay the majority of (or all) program costs, and have the lion's share of authority and responsibility in determining program direction. Academic researchers may, of course, be involved in such programs, but they are quite likely to follow a participatory action research ideal, in which the professional researcher's profile is much lower than in the disease prevention research programs of the first type.

Ottawa Charter
for Health Promotion

The Ottawa Charter for Health Promotion is a very important milestone in the development of the health promotion ideology that underlies health promotion via community development (WHO, 1986). The charter, a political document, defines *health promotion* as the process of enabling people to take control over, and to improve, their health. As will be described in more detail in the second part of this chapter, the Ottawa Charter was the crest of a wave that had been building for years, based on actions in many countries. It has been followed and bolstered by succeeding waves leading to landmark international conferences on health promotion in Adelaide, Australia (1988), Sundsvall, Sweden (1991), and Jakarta, Indonesia (1997). Together, these have had a definitive influence on the development and shaping of a coordinated and determined international, politically based movement that bears the flag of health promotion and that has community development principles at its core.

At the communitywide level, the best known "face" of this movement is the World Health Organization's (WHO's) Healthy Cities Project, in which over 1,000 cities worldwide have started the process of shaping healthier public policy (Ashton, 1992). The successes of Healthy Cities have helped spawn a number of other projects that have worldwide reach, such as Health Promoting Schools, Workplaces, Hospitals, and Islands programs. At the same time, the project has done much to help us understand the barriers to research in such initiatives. Healthy Cities has thus been chosen as the exemplar of this program type.

Cardiovascular Disease Prevention

Starting in Finland and in the United States in 1972 with the North Karelia Project and the Stanford Three Community Study, many cardiovascular disease prevention projects have since been carried out at the communitywide level, on every continent, in dozens of countries, and in hundreds of towns and cities (Farquhar, Maccoby, & Wood, 1985; Puska, 1988; Shea & Basch, 1990). Much of the earliest activity was centered in Europe, with the program in Finland, of course, but also with programs in both (then) Germanys, Hungary, Italy, Norway, Switzerland, Yugoslavia, and the U.S.S.R. (Puska, 1988).

INITIAL FINDINGS

The initial progress reports from the European projects and California were electrifyingly positive (Farquhar, Maccoby, Wood, Alexander, et al., 1977; Maccoby, Farquhar, Wood, & Alexander, 1977; Puska, 1988; Puska, Nissinen, et al., 1985; Puska, Tuomilehto, Salonen, et al., 1981; Salonen, Puska, & Mustaaniemi, 1979). The cities and towns that were approached were eager to participate. Community organization models that had been developed for other applications worked well in the new CVD prevention programs (Rothman, 1979). Interventions that were grounded in communications and behavior change theories could be implemented at the communitywide level. Early trends in behavior and risk factors favored the hypothesis that the community-based approach to CVD reduction was feasible.

The early reports of success helped stimulate the development of and provide the resources needed to launch a new generation of very large-scale community-based CVD prevention research and demonstration projects in the United States, in California (Farquhar, 1978), Rhode Island (Lasater et al., 1984), and Minnesota (Blackburn et al., 1984). Although the three new American projects were independently conceived, their research methodologies were developed in collaboration, resulting in an unprecedented level of comparability that was to prove invaluable in later analyses (Flora et al., 1993; Stone, 1991; Winkleby, Feldman, & Murray, 1997).

These new American projects began to implement community-based intervention during the early 1980s, and reports of early experiences published by the mid-1980s added to the excitement generated by the first-generation projects (Farquhar, Maccoby, & Wood, 1985; Lasater et al., 1984; Mittelmark, Luepker, et al., 1986). In the public health field, strong enthusiasm developed for the community-based approach to health promotion pioneered by the CVD prevention projects. This was understandable, as both in Europe and North America the exemplar projects were conducted using primarily a medical/epidemiological/public health approach that was familiar and comfortable to public health workers and the public.

The basic approach combined population-based risk factor reduction education with medical treatment of those at particularly high risk, using a broad mix of behavioral, social change, and community organization models (Blackburn, 1992; Farquhar, Maccoby, & Wood, 1985; Kottke, Puska, Salonen, Tuomilehto, & Nissinen, 1985; Loken, Swim, & Mittelmark, 1990; Puska, 1988; Rose, 1992). The Finnish and the large-scale American projects had risk behavior and factor change (smoking, diet composition, blood pressure, blood cholesterol, physical activity, body weight) as primary objectives and aimed as well to reduce CVD morbidity and mortality rates.

RESEARCH METHODS

The evaluation designs of these exemplar projects attempted to emulate the gold standard experiment design as far as possible, but practical and financial limitations resulted in weak designs in practice. Comparing communities exposed to special interventions with communities not exposed to special interventions was a common feature, but there were very few communities enrolled, and there was no randomization.

These projects were not, in fact, experiments at all. They followed much more closely the model of quasiexperimental designs introduced by Campbell and Stanley (1963), but even as quasiexperimental designs, they were weak, lacking the multiple control groups needed to control for various biases introduced by sampling methods, lacking randomization, and displaying other design weaknesses. However, it was believed that strong effects of education programs could be obtained and detected even with relatively weak study designs. More to the point, strong experimental designs with many units of analysis, control groups, and random assignment were not affordable or practical (Kottke, 1995).

EXEMPLARS

These four projects, among the many conducted, are singled out here for close examination. That is because they have been held out by many workers in health promotion as exemplar projects, representing the highest state of the art of community-based disease prevention research. Their approach to study design, to community, to intervention, and to measurement has been widely emulated. Scientific reviewers, funding agencies, and journal editors have employed these four exemplar projects as yardsticks against which to measure the adequacy of other community-based disease prevention initiatives.

MAIN FINDINGS

Now, 25 and more years after the start of the first of these programs, the main results, those related to long-term risk factor change and to morbidity and mortality change, are available in the published scientific literature, and to many they are confusing.

Looking first to Europe and the North Karelia Project, the main objective at the outset of the project was to achieve a substantial decline in CVD mortality, especially among middle-aged men (Puska, Tuomilehto, Vartiainen, Korhonen, & Torppa, 1995). Coronary heart disease mortality in all of Finland was tracked over a 20-year period, beginning in the early 1970s. Beginning with rates that were among the highest in the world, there was a remarkable decline in CHD death rates, greater than 50%, over the next 20 years. In North Karelia (the intervention community), the decline in CHD deaths was even steeper during the decade after intervention was launched. There were also significant declines in some risk factors, providing the earliest evidence that the community-based strategy worked (Puska, Nissinen, et al., 1985).

However, by the early 1980s, the rest of Finland had caught up with North Karelia. By the last year of the study, 1992, the decline in CVD mortality in men from the preprogram period was 57% in North Karelia and 52% in all Finland (Puska, Tuomilehto, Variainen, et al., 1995), a difference of only 5%. The complete story of the North Karelia experience with mortality change is, of course, much more complicated than can be summarized here. There was, for example, a decline in cancer mortality in North Karelia that was larger and more sustained than in all Finland during the 20 years of the project (Puska, Tuomilehto, Variainen, et al., 1995).

It is important to note, however, that North Karelia was the first project to observe a pattern of findings that was to be repeated in the other exemplar projects. This was a pattern of strong secular trends (also called temporal trends: changes occurring over a long period of time) of reduced risk factors and CVD rates and early success of intervention in accelerating the favorable trends but, eventually, a diminished and statistically nonsignificant difference between the secular trend effect and the intervention effect.

Looking next to the three American studies, the Stanford Five City Project's 6-year risk reduction program yielded mixed findings over the long term, based on comparisons between the project's intervention communities and control communities. Among women, there were significant or near-significant differences in the expected direction between intervention and control communities for knowledge of cardiovascular diseases and for coronary heart disease risk. But significant differences were not observed for blood pressure, total cholesterol, smoking, body mass index, and all-cause mortality risk (Winkleby, Taylor, Jatulis, & Fortmann, 1996).

Among men in the Stanford study, there were significant differences between intervention and control communities in the hypothesized direction in knowledge of cardiovascular diseases, systolic blood pressure, diastolic blood pressure, and body mass index. But no significant differences were seen for total cholesterol, smoking, coronary heart disease risk, and all-cause mortality risk (Winkleby et al., 1996).

As a general finding, the control communities improved during the course of the study, as did the intervention communities. The greatest differences between intervention and control communities were observed at the end of 6 years of intervention, but these differences had begun to fade 4 to 5 years after the formal intervention ended, a pattern similar to that observed in North Karelia.

The Stanford researchers concluded that although some sustained effects were observed, the modest net differences in risk factors suggested the need for better study designs and better interventions to accelerate positive risk factor change risk (Winkleby et al., 1996).

In the Pawtucket, Rhode Island, program, after 7 years of intervention, there was a significant difference between the intervention and control communities in the expected direction for body mass index only. There were, as well, improvements favoring the treatment community at the peak of intervention in smoking and cardiovascular risk, but these improvements faded after intervention was ended. There were no significant differences after the conclusion of intervention between the intervention and control communities for total cholesterol, systolic blood pressure, diastolic blood pressure, smoking, and cardiovascular disease risk (Carleton et al., 1995). Thus the pattern described earlier for the North Karelia and Stanford projects was observed also in the Pawtucket project.

The Pawtucket researchers concluded that achieving cardiovascular risk reduction at the community level was feasible, but maintaining statistically significant differences between the treatment and the control communities was not. Thus, the project provided only limited evidence for the feasibility of cardiovascular disease risk reduction by the community-based education approach (Carleton et al., 1995).

The Minnesota Heart Health Program's three intervention and three control communities provided the most powerful test (statistically speaking) of the community-based approach to CVD prevention. The intensive intervention phase lasted 5 to 6 years, depending on the community (Mittelmark, Luepker, et al., 1986). Early results were positive, based on findings from successive cross-sectional surveys. Within 2 to 3 years of the beginning of intervention, the control communities had greater exposure to CVD prevention messages than at the beginning of the study, but the intervention communities had significantly greater exposure that seemed attributable to the special education program (Luepker, Murray, et al., 1994). A similar positive pattern was seen for total blood cholesterol, systolic and diastolic blood pressure, body mass index, and physical activity. For cigarette smoking, the trend among women favored the intervention by the midpoint of the education program, but among men no difference between intervention and control communities was observed.

Despite the early signs of success, the Minnesota program's results at the end of the intervention phase were very similar to the pattern already described for North Karelia, Stanford, and Pawtucket. The initial improvement over the favorable secular trend that was observed in the intervention communities was not sustained, and at the end of the intervention, the risk profiles of the intervention and control communities were almost indistinguishable. The sole exception was cigarette smoking among women, for which the early trend favoring the intervention communities was maintained over the longer term (Luepker, Murray, et al., 1994).

The only one of the three large American studies that has as yet published morbidity and mortality results is the Minnesota project, and these findings are, not surprisingly, consistent with the risk factor results. Coronary heart disease rates decreased in the control communities during the course of the study and the treatment communities did not differ significantly from the secular trend (Luepker, Råstam, et al., 1996).

The Minnesota researchers concluded that many of the interventions were effective in targeted groups within the intervention communities. But against the backdrop of strong secular trends of declining risk factors, the program effects were modest in size and duration and generally were within chance levels (Luepker, Murray, et al., 1994).

JOINT ANALYSES

Finally, from these American studies, good collaboration between the research teams enabled a joint analysis to be undertaken, in which the six intervention communities of Stanford, Pawtucket, and Minnesota were compared with the six control communities with regard to risk factors and coronary heart disease mortality risk. The joint analysis of these data revealed that for most risk factors, exposure to intervention improved the risk factor profile in comparison to the control group, but these improvements never reached a statistically significant level (Winkleby, Feldman, et al., 1997).

WHAT HAPPENED?

The authors of these studies and others have of course given much thought to the puzzling pattern of findings. In all the intervention communities in these exemplar studies, the intervention program was welcomed and many citizens contributed time and effort to assist the programs in reaching their goals. Education was launched in schools, worksites, community settings such as groceries and restaurants, screening centers, and churches. Community organization approaches were common to all the studies.

Program evaluations of these components showed in many cases that the programs reached their intended audience and had their intended effects (Flora et al., 1993; Helakorpi & Puska, 1995; Mittelmark, Hunt, et al., 1996). Education was sustained for 5 years or more, and many citizens had multiple educational contacts with the program in their community. The communities, in other words, embraced the interventions, which were intensive and extensive. These successes stimulated other researchers and other communities in many countries to adopt the community-based approach to CVD prevention pioneered by the exemplars. Well before the risk factor and morbidity and mortality results were available, the community-based approach was recommended as an effective prevention mechanism for public health (Elder, Schmid, Dower, & Hedlund, 1993; Schwartz et al., 1993).

Based on surveys of the populations living in the control areas, the secular risk factor trends showed improvement. The degree to which this was so was not expected when the studies were planned. Nevertheless, in the early stages it seemed that the intervention communities were doing significantly better than the control communities. Yet, in the final analysis, the main objectives of these studies were not achieved. Risk factors did not on the whole differ between intervention and control communities, and all communities tended to show improvement. The more limited data on morbidity and mortality are consistent with the overall pattern described here.

CRITIQUE

Critical analysis of these experiences has not resulted in clear-cut consensus about what happened. Some analysts believe that the data, viewed in a broad perspective, support a conclusion that community-based programs can change heart disease rates (Kottke, 1995). The core of this argument is that the studies were conducted in the context of nationwide community intervention. This took the form of national CVD education campaigns, publicity about tobacco and public health warnings, and news reports about the many clinical trials that attempted to show experimentally that intervention was effective. The consumer products industries made product changes to keep up with the changing health values of the public. Thus, despite the results of the research programs, the community-based approach is to be recommended based on broader experiences with the approach (Kottke, 1995). Bolstering this argument are the positive results of many studies of specific intervention components that have already been described.

There are others who take a skeptical stand on the issue. They view the risk factor and morbidity and mortality data from the research projects at face value and conclude that the communitywide, education-based strategy for CVD is not the optimal approach (McCormick & Skrabanek, 1988; Syme, 1997).

However, it seems difficult and even inappropriate to pass a simple judgment on these studies or on the approach they have pioneered. The community-based CVD prevention research projects tested not just a single, main hypothesis, but rather aimed to test many interrelated hypotheses and probe many research questions. Is it possible to attract the attention, energy, and resources of communities to work for CVD prevention? Will diverse sectors (business, medicine, education, public health, etc.) cross barriers and work together? Can communitywide health promotion be combined with rigorous outcome research? Can education programs compete successfully with existing marketing and advertising forces? Can medical services be reoriented to include serious prevention efforts? Does the experience of working for CVD prevention strengthen a community's ability to deal with other challenges that may arise? Can the processes through which community-based CVD prevention programs are implemented be traced, understood, and replicated?

Many hundreds of scientific papers from the CVD prevention studies on these themes are to be found in the published literature, and key references have been given above. Succinctly put, the answers to the questions about the feasibility of implementing and maintaining communitywide programs for CVD prevention are almost uniformly positive. Questions about the effectiveness of specific educational programs have yielded mixed results, but many proven interventions have been documented. The answers regarding program effects on risk factors and disease are almost uniformly negative, viewed over the long term.

Why is this so? What can we learn from this perplexing pattern of outcomes? How can these experiences be used to improve our ability to implement more effective community-based disease prevention programs? At least five possible explanations deserve attention:

> The education programs themselves were ineffective.
> The surveys and measurement methods were inadequate.
> Strong secular changes overwhelmed the studies.
> Effect size estimates were too optimistic.
> The study designs were poor.
> The conceptual basis of the exemplars' approach is ill founded.

Education Programs

The obvious question of the effectiveness of the educational programs themselves has been examined (Carleton et al., 1995; Fortmann et al., 1995; Luepker et al., 1994). If the education offered to the public was poor quality, not able to produce the intended effects, a plausible explanation for the lack of effect on risk factors and morbidity and mortality would be at hand. However, this possibility does not stand up well to examination. In many small-scale studies within the intervention communities, program effectiveness was measured in selected target groups, children in schools, for example. Many components of the intervention were demonstrated to be effective (Mittelmark, Hunt, et al., 1993). That this was so is supported by the general finding, already described here, of behavior and risk factor changes in the anticipated direction during the early years of the intervention programs.

Survey and Data Analysis Methods

Inaccurate survey data and/or poor analysis methods could be suspected as at least a partial cause of the pattern of findings that are so perplexing. However, this explanation, too, does not stand up well to examination. Experienced research teams were responsible for the projects. The projects received very close peer scrutiny for scientific quality before they were approved to proceed. Rigorous quality control measures were put into place to oversee data collection. Experienced statisticians performed the data analyses. The quality of the work overall has been critically examined in the peer review process that precedes publication in scientific journals.

There were, of course, errors made in these projects. Error in research is unavoidable. But errors were prevented to the extent possible and dealt with straightforwardly when detected. It does not seem plausible that lack of rigor in the survey and data analysis aspects of the studies can explain the results.

Secular Trends and Effect Sizes

The strong secular changes favoring improved health-related behavior, lowered risk factors, and reduced CVD morbidity and mortality were not anticipated (Carleton et al., 1995; Fortmann et al., 1995; Luepker, Murray, et al., 1994; Luepker, Råstam, et al., 1996; Murray et al., 1994; Winkleby et al., 1996). Very few data on CVD trends were available when these studies were in the planning stages.

In fact, in the United States, smoking trends were already improving by the time the American studies were launched and national education campaigns on blood pressure, cholesterol, and smoking were in the planning stages or already launched. Also, the social, political, and scientific climate that permitted such large, expensive undertakings to be launched indicated a strong and widespread interest in the possibility of reducing population risk for CVD rather than only treating its end results.

Had the secular trends for strong improvement in CVD risk behaviors, risk factors, and morbidity and mortality been appreciated at the time these studies were first contemplated, it is doubtful whether they would have been designed as they were. Improving secular trends cause researchers severe difficulties with regard to both intervention and measurement. Even the most intensive special intervention can expect at best only to borrow from future improvements that will arrive with or without special intervention (Carleton et al., 1995).

This goes a long way, perhaps, to explaining the encouraging but temporary improvements that all the intervention communities experienced during the course of intervention. Future community-based research for disease prevention should be preceded by sufficient descriptive research so that secular trends are well described and understood beforehand (Murray, 1995). They should not proceed unless they have good reason to believe that their special intervention will produce a significant health gain over and above that to be expected based on the secular trend (Murray, 1995). As the epidemiologist Susser (1995) has poetically written, small effects nestling under the wings of large ones are difficult to elicit. If the secular trend is improving, the decision to proceed or not with a special intervention should include careful consideration of the borrowing-from-the-future phenomenon.

This is not to say that speeding a population's improving health is not a good idea, only that the cost should be weighed against the realistic health gain. This is not an issue for researchers to grapple with alone. Community-based disease prevention research depends very much on community resources, and the community should be a full and well-informed partner in this decision making. Practically, this means that the frequent practice of recruiting communities to research projects after the funding has been obtained should change. The informed consent of the community should be obtained before research funding is sought. The informed consent should include due consideration to possible positive effects, negative effects, null effects, and unexpected effects.

Community-based research under conditions of improving secular trends encounters serious measurement problems, in addition to the intervention problems discussed above. Imagine a proven intervention X of known treatment effect and another proven intervention Y, with the same treatment effect. The difference between X and Y is that X produces its effect more quickly than does Y. These two are pitted against each other in a communitywide research study with two communities that are equivalent initially with respect to the outcome variable.

In the simplest study design, with one measurement at the beginning of the study and one at the end, the more rapid effect of X will not be discovered. Considered graphically, the intercepts and slopes of the lines depicting change in the outcome variable will be the same for X and Y. The only way to detect the special, rapid effect of X is to conduct many more surveys, to capture the point, extent, and duration of X's departure from Y.

Now substitute for Y the "natural" treatment of an improving secular trend in a control community, and the implications for the communitywide trial study design are obvious. When secular trends are worsening or stable, fewer repeated surveys are needed, reducing cost and complexity. When secular trends are improving, frequent repeated surveys are required, increasing cost and complexity.

This adds weight to the argument that communitywide disease prevention research should be launched early in the genesis of a public health problem, ideally, when the problem is still a growing one. The research will be less costly, the peak magnitude of the problem might well be blunted, and the net gain to the public's health will be enhanced.

That is the ideal. The reality is that the social, political, and scientific processes that prepare the ground for community-based intervention research unfold typically over a long time period (Koepsell, Diehr, Cheadle, & Kristal, 1995). In the United States, the major community-based CVD prevention studies were started years after the U.S. Surgeon General and the public became alarmed about tobacco. Major clinical studies on the causes and prevention of CVD had already been publicized. When the American studies started, their intervention and control communities had already experienced newspaper articles and television programs on healthy lifestyles. American business was already producing alternative products that appealed to the health conscious. The service industry had already established a pattern of rapid expansion in the number of health and fitness facilities. Lifestyle modification for improved health was already well on the way to becoming a major fad.

Clearly, it is to be desired that society react rapidly because, inevitably, new public health problems develop. A fundamental requirement for such rapid reaction is a public health surveillance mechanism that gives early warning. Another fundamental requirement is a research establishment that has the inclination, the skills, and the resources to work rapidly with communities to develop effective intervention in response to early warning. A third fundamental requirement is political will to react positively and quickly when new public health problems surface. Finally, a health promotion infrastructure is needed that connects national resources with local resources, to ensure that proven interventions are disseminated rapidly and wisely.

Study Design

The discussions about secular trend and effect size are tied up in a larger issue, that of the study design itself. As already mentioned, the study designs of the major CVD prevention research projects were inspired by the classic experimental design (Susser, 1995). But, lacking randomization, multiple control groups, and large sample sizes, these scaled-up designs are weak (Carleton et al., 1995; Fortmann et al., 1995; Murray et al., 1994; Winkleby et al., 1996).

The problem of scale is particularly well appreciated in the philosophy of design, both structural and biological. An important and basic principle of scale discovered by Galileo is that as a structure is scaled up, the weight of the structure increases as a cube of the dimensions, so that a doubling of size, for example, results in an eight-fold weight increase (Gordon, 1978). This principle has been cited as a prime limiting factor in the size of animals, as an example of a practical consequence of the scaling problem (Gordon, 1978).

An important consequence of this principle is that a design that functions well is limited in the degree to which it can be scaled up and still function as intended. Scaling down can also present problems for the function of a design. The example of a catapult (to call upon an unfortunate martial metaphor) illustrates the problem nicely. A catapult of the right size to breach an enemy's defenses cannot be scaled up or down without sacrifices. Scaled down to a convenient pocket model, its mechanical function may be perfect, but its effect on enemy defenses will be negligible. Scaled up to a magnificent size with the theoretical capability of crushing a fortress with a single blow, its huge weight would likely prohibit its movement from the protected place of construction to the fortunate target fortress.

Similarly, the scaled-up experimental design requires sacrifices. The essence of the experimental design, control with randomization, is usually the first sacrifice. When very few units are available for randomization, the likelihood of achieving preexperimental equivalence in experimental and control groups is lowered. As a result, randomization is usually abandoned in favor of selecting communities for assignment to condition based on convenience factors, as was the case for the exemplar CVD prevention studies. Aside from practical considerations, lack of randomization opens a trial to criticism, whichever way the results turn out (Koepsell et al., 1995).

Because the unit of analysis should be at the same level as the unit of intervention, and these numbers are typically very small, large standard errors for the estimates of treatment effects are to be expected, and statistical power to detect the effect of interest is poor (Murray, 1995).

Further, community-level interventions are composed typically of many components, but the desirable component analysis that would require many control groups is not feasible because too few study units are available to create the needed control groups. It is thus not possible to credit the effective components, discredit the ineffective ones, or know the effect of a given component in the absence of all the other components (Koepsell et al., 1995; Mittelmark, Hunt, et al., 1993).

Finally, it might well be that very strong effects will be detected in even a weak study design. But there is little to suggest that strong effects should be expected in community-based disease prevention research (Susser, 1995). Taken together, the complexities of secular trends, relatively small effect sizes, and problems of scale advise extreme caution when contemplating a communitywide trial design (Fortmann et al., 1995; Mittelmark, Hunt, et al., 1993).

Some have argued that the communitywide trial design should not be abandoned but, rather, strengthened, particularly by including many more communities than has been typical and employing random assignment, as is done in true experiments. Unfortunately, even these major improvements may prove to be insufficient. A most instructive case study of this approach is the Community Intervention Trial for Smoking Cessation (COMMIT), which aimed to improve on the design weaknesses of previous community studies (Gail, Byar, Pechacek, & Corle, 1992). Twenty-two communities (at the town and city level) in North America were selected for involvement with randomization to intervention or control conditions occurring in 1988. An intervention protocol was developed so that each intervention community implemented the intervention in as similar a manner as community differences would allow.

The intervention was, by any measure, extensive and intensive (Glasgow et al., 1996). The United States' National Cancer Institute financially and scientifically backed the experiment. The resources available to the study were most luxurious by international standards.

To make effect assessment as straightforward as possible, the main outcome measure was simply the cessation rate among smokers, of which more than 20,000 were tracked. The study concluded in 1993. The data analysis that followed was extraordinarily thoughtful (Green, Corle, et al., 1995).

In other words, the financial backing, planning, study design, intervention, and analysis of COMMIT were very close to as good as a communitywide trial could possibly be (Susser, 1995). Yet, the results must be considered disappointing indeed. Over the course of the project, there was no intervention effect on heavy smoking prevalence, and overall smoking prevalence decreased 3.5 percentage points in intervention communities, compared to 3.2 percentage points in control communities, an insignificant difference (COMMIT Research Group, 1995). The researchers cited the improving secular trend as an important factor in the outcome.

Emerging Perspectives. There are alternatives to continuing up the path of weightier community-level trials. The Stanford group in the United States is very experienced with the community trial design, having conducted two such studies, the Three-Community Study and the Five-Community Study. Their counsel is straightforward, and in clear concert with the lessons that have been discussed here:

> The emphasis of future studies should shift from whether community-wide change is possible to improving methods of community organization and health education, reaching diverse sub-populations that are at high risk, incorporating ongoing efforts into health care and other social structures, instituting and maintaining regulatory and environmental changes that enhance the effects of health education, and improving the monitoring of chronic disease risk and incidence. There is an urgent need to understand communities better, particularly how communities differ in health status and in their readiness and resources to change health status. Clearly, communities change over time, but the forces that drive this change are far from understood. (Fortmann et al., 1995)

The Stanford group is not alone in raising a flag of caution. A central figure in the North Karelia Project, Pekka Puska, has not only questioned the feasibility of random allocation of whole communities, but also pointed out that the community intervention trial design may contradict the true nature of community organization (Puska, 1995a, 1995b). Furthermore, the Pawtucket Heart Health Program researchers in the United States have concluded that the effectiveness of CVD prevention may require a strategy that goes well beyond community, including integration of efforts at the community, state or province, and national levels to affect policies, milieu, and practices (Carleton et al., 1995).

Conceptual Basis of Communitywide CVD Prevention Research

For the most part, the criticisms noted here emerge from practical concerns about the feasibility of doing good science in the framework of the communitywide trial design. It is useful also to consider the theoretical basis for the community-based trial design and ask what implications the experiences of the exemplars have for the theory. The core theoretical framework upon which these studies have been constructed cannot be attributed to any one source, but Rose must be credited with "pulling it all together" in the very accessible volume *The Strategy of Preventive Medicine* (Rose, 1992). The basic premises are these:

Risk factors for a large number of diseases and health problems are distributed in populations in a graded manner.

There is often no obvious and clinically meaningful risk factor threshold that differentiates those at risk and those not at risk for a chronic disease.

For many chronic diseases, there are many more people in a population at a relatively moderate level of risk than at the highest levels of risk.

Addressing only the very high risk (clinically recognized) segment of a population misses the opportunity to improve the risk profile of the entire population.

Modest risk lowering among many persons with moderate risk factor levels will shift the risk factor profile of the entire population in a favorable manner.

A populationwide approach to intervention is thus called for, the objectives of which should be to reduce the average level of the population's risk through intervention for all and to intervene intensively for those few at the highest level of risk.

The theory is not specific about how the population is to be specified, or about what kinds of interventions are called for. However, for the epidemiologists and other public health researchers that subscribe to this theoretical perspective, the geopolitical unit *city/town* has, for practical reasons, been the population unit of choice for the trials that are needed to test the theory. Cities and towns of good size are large enough to function as "epidemiological communities" for CVD prevention studies. Populations in the 10 to 100s of thousands are needed for the epidemiological surveillance of risk factor and morbidity and mortality changes over a reasonable period of time.

From an intervention standpoint, cities and towns seem at face value to be "natural" intervention units. A city or town is united by many common social, political, and physical structures—local government, schools, workplaces, radio stations, newspapers, shopping facilities, parks, roads, and so on. Thus, in theory at least, the city or town has seemed a reasonable choice as the unit to be assigned to intervention or control conditions.

As already described here, much experience shows that, indeed, intervention at this organizational level is feasible and desirable. Many people identify with the town they live in, they are willing to work with each other to improve the quality of life of the community, and they have experience in group problem solving. As several following chapters demonstrate, the community approach to health promotion requires adaptation that depends on project aims and local conditions. However, when adapted properly, the approach seems well suited to a remarkable range of problems and local conditions.

Nevertheless, a rigorous test of the population-based strategy seems to be impractical, on the basis of the lessons discussed above. The main conclusion arrived at here is not that community-wide health promotion is inadvisable, but rather that research at the communitywide level of analysis should be undertaken only when the obstacles discussed above can be overcome. This may be possible in some countries with large populations and many communities, especially for problems with worsening secular trends. Tobacco use in the People's Republic of China comes to mind as a prime example (Chen, Xu, Collins, Li, & Peto, 1997). However, given the enormous resources that are required to mount and conduct such trials, the communitywide trial design will be very difficult to justify even when the conditions are right.

There are viable alternative approaches that do not depend on the communitywide trial study design. One approach is to define *community* at the level of settings such as schools, workplaces, and churches, for example. At this level of analysis, the challenges that face a community trial design are conceptually the same as encountered by the communitywide design but may be easier to overcome. Schools, in particular, have been settings for successful health promotion research projects in many countries, and today there exists a worldwide network of practitioners and researchers that continue to develop this strategy (WHO, 1997).

Another approach is to maintain the communitywide perspective on health promotion action within a research framework that does not require a communitywide trial design. The research questions that fit in such a framework are plentiful. Many of the most interesting have to do with core community development processes (Rothman, 1996). How can we improve methods of community organization and achieve better partnership with communities? How can a community's own assets be best applied to solving its health challenges? How can we provide expert guidance and at the same time respect community expertise? How can we improve the short- and long-term effectiveness of specific intervention components? What are the important processes that are universal to effective community health promotion? How can the community approach to health promotion be better adapted to the cultural diversities of communities in different parts of the world? How can the basic determinants of health be better promoted, including safe environment, education, employment, and freedom of choice?

A number of these questions obviously have much to do with the core ideas of community development, which are centered on increasing the capacities and employing the resources of communities to address a broad range of current and future issues and challenges that they themselves identify as important. We move now to this theme.

Community Development Approaches

Communitywide health promotion programs that use a community development approach have evolved from a very different perspective than did the disease prevention projects discussed in the first part of this chapter. Disease prevention programs have clearly identifiable roots in preventive medicine, public health, health education, and social psychology. These are professional and academic fields. Community trials on the practice of disease prevention have been designed, implemented, and monitored by interdisciplinary teams who work with communities to solve problems that have been identified by the health professionals. In other words, the "engine" pulling disease prevention is professional.

The community development approach to health promotion is less easy to characterize. The term *community development* has been in use a long time and has taken on many shades of meaning. Other labels are in use that can be confused with community development, such as community mobilization, community empowerment, community action, community organization, and community-based programming, even though community development workers view their approach as distinct (Ploeg et al., 1996). Much of community development has the goal of reducing inequity, especially poverty, but the range of challenges to which the approach is applied is truly remarkable, including rural economic development, school lunch programs, community cultural development, encouraging citizen participation in local politics, building problem-solving partnerships that bridge traditional boundaries within communities, improved housing, jobs programs, and, of course, health promotion—and these are but a few examples.

Whatever the issue to which it is applied, what is common to almost all community development initiatives is a philosophy and process that (a) emphasizes the participation of people in their own development (as opposed to the "client" state), (b) recognizes and uses people's assets (as opposed to attending mainly to their problems and limitations), (c) encourages the participation of people in the generation of information about community needs and assets (as opposed to research controlled by professionals), (d) empowers people to make choices (as opposed to the management of people by institutions of power), and (e) involves people in the political processes that affect their lives (as opposed to nonparticipation) (Brown, 1991; Campfens, 1997; Dluhy & Kravitz, 1990; Fawcett et al., 1995; Green, George, et al., 1995; Kretzmann & McKnight, 1997; Labonte, 1993; Perkins & Zimmerman, 1995; Schulz, Israel, Zimmerman, & Checkoway, 1995).

In other words, the engine pulling community development is the people themselves—at least in theory. A (manageable) tension in the philosophy of community development is that community development ideas, writings, methods, conferences, and journals are the work and activity mostly of academics and professionals, just as is the case for disease prevention. Such professionals serve obviously critical roles as catalysts, advisers, leaders, developers, and doers (Rohde, Chatterjee, & Morley, 1993). Although community development work rarely springs directly from the grassroots, untended by trained professionals, community development takes the fundamental view that community capacity building to enable local leadership is a vital element in the community development process (Hawe, Noort, King, & Jordens, 1997; Jackson, Mitchell, & Wright, 1989.

HEALTHY CITIES

Healthy Cities is a health promotion application of the community development approach, although critics could argue easily that a program designed and promoted by the World Health Organization, an instrument of governments, skates at or over the edge of the ideal (Lupton, 1995, p. 59). Be that as it may, much has been learned about communitywide health promotion practice and research through Healthy Cities (Duhl, 1996; Flynn, 1996). To appreciate these lessons requires some familiarity with the historical, mostly political, developments that led to the Healthy Cities project.

Few would disagree that 1974 was the seminal year and Canada the seminal place in the genesis of the community development approach to health promotion. That was the year the Canadian Department of Health and Welfare issued the report *A New Perspective on the Health of Canadians*, signaling what many have called the "era of health promotion" (Lalonde, 1974). The report stated that improved health of populations had more to do with improving social and environmental conditions than with advances in medical science and access to medical care. The report suggested the setting of national health goals and pointed to health promotion as an important new strategy. In 1976, The Health Promotion Directorate was established in Canada, providing the beginnings of a health promotion infrastructure that integrated public and private sectors at the local community, region, and national levels.

In 1977, the Thirtieth World Health Assembly of the WHO, stimulated in good part by Canada's model, laid the foundation for worldwide health promotion community development initiatives with its declaration that "the main social targets of governments and WHO in the coming decades should be the attainment by all citizens of the world by the year 2000 of a level of health that will permit them to lead a socially and economically productive life" (WHO, 1993, p. 1). This was the beginning of a campaign that became known as "Health for All by the Year 2000." This set the stage for a key development in 1978, when the WHO and UNICEF adopted the Alma-Alta Declaration (Alma-Alta, U.S.S.R.), which identified individual and community education as essential elements of primary health care. Also that year, the Toronto Board of Health issued its report *Public Health in the 1980's*, the Lalonde Report of municipal public health.

The period 1984 to 1986 was pivotal. The idea for the Healthy Cities project was conceived at a workshop in Canada called "Health Toronto 2000," which brought together a wide variety of community sectors and interest groups to explore ways to make Toronto a healthier city (Draper, Curtice, Hooper, & Goumans, 1993). The Canadian Public Health Association held a conference that included one of the first formal presentations on the healthy city concept (Duhl, 1985). The member states of the WHO European Region adopted a set of 38 European targets for health. Statistical indicators for monitoring progress toward the Health for All targets were adopted. The Targets for Health developed by the European Office of WHO in 1984 were published, translated into 19 languages, and distributed worldwide.

In 1986, the first International Conference on Health Promotion was held in Ottawa, Canada, culminating in the adoption of the Ottawa Charter for Health Promotion. The charter was crafted as a brief, accessible, political manifesto. At its core is the contention that health is a resource for everyday life, not an end in itself. The charter identifies conditions and resources for health, including peace, shelter, education, food, income, a stable ecosystem, sustainable resources, social justice, and equity. It states that improvement in health requires a secure foundation in these basic prerequisites. It identifies health promotion as the process of enabling people to increase control over, and to improve, their health and states that health promotion is not just the responsibility of the health sector. The charter identifies three main health promotion strategies, including political advocacy, action to reduce inequity and enable people to reach their fullest health potential, and coordinated action involving all elements and sectors of society rather just the health care sector alone.

The charter recommends action in five arenas: the building of healthy public policy, the creation of supportive environments, the empowerment of communities, the development of personal skills so people can make informed choices, and a reorientation of health services to better incorporate health promotion practice, research, and teaching (the full text of the charter is available via the Internet at http://www.who.dk/policy/ottawa.htm).

The charter, which was ultimately translated into more than 40 languages, has been very influential, especially in Europe, where several Eastern and Central European countries have reorganized their health care systems to incorporate health promotion ideas at the core. But the charter is also a controversial document, with at least one critic going so far as to pronounce its definition of health promotion as merely banal (Seedhouse, 1997, p. 33). Critics aside, the developments that culminated in the Ottawa Charter set the stage for a major test of health promotion, WHO-style, called Healthy Cities.

Healthy Cities: Aims

Healthy Cities was conceived as a means of testing virtually all the elements of the Ottawa Charter at the community level. At a meeting of representatives of 21 European cities in Lisbon in 1986, the initiative was developed around five major aims (Ashton, 1992, p. 8). First, the cities would develop action-based health plans following the framework of Health for All, the health promotion principles of the Ottawa Charter, and the 38 European targets for health. Second, the cities would develop "models of good practice" to illustrate the key principles of health promotion. Such models could then be disseminated to other communities. Third, the cities would monitor program activities and conduct research on the effectiveness of the models of good practice. Fourth, the cities would collaborate to disseminate ideas and experiences. Fifth, the cities would foster mutual support, learning, and cultural exchange between the cities and towns of Europe.

To achieve these aims, the initiative developed a seven-part strategy (Ashton, 1992). They would establish an intersectional group of community decision makers to develop an overview of health in the community and "unlock" their organizations to work with each other at all levels. The cities would establish a technical support group to work on collaborative analysis and planning. They would conduct a community diagnosis down to the small-area level, with an emphasis on health inequalities and the public's perceptions of the community and its health. The cities would establish links with educational institutions, develop these into teaching and research partnerships, and work together to identify appropriate urban health indicators. All agencies involved in the Healthy Cities initiative would assess the health promotion potential of their organizations, develop health impact statements to make the potential for improvement explicit, and map assets for health. The cities would stimulate public debate and discussion about health in the city, within organizations and in the local mass media. The cities would implement interventions to achieve Health for All objectives and monitor and evaluate the interventions.

Formal Establishment of the Healthy Cities Project

At the beginning of 1987, 11 European cities became the founding members of the WHO Healthy Cities Project, coordinated from WHO's European Regional office in Copenhagen. The original network of 11 cities expanded by 14 more within a year. By 1992, barely 5 years after its start, the Healthy Cities network had grown to over 500 cities in Europe and 300 cities in other parts of the world (Tsouros, 1995). As of this writing, more than 1,000 cities participate (the latest information about Healthy Cities is available via the Internet at http://www.who.ch/peh/hlthcit/ index.htm).

Healthy Cities: Methods

Healthy Cities in Europe operates on three levels. An international network of project cities with strong political commitment has the task of developing new approaches to health promotion and tests their feasibility. Within each country, the project cities establish links with other communities, serving as resources in national and subnational networks. Healthy Cities national and international networks stay in contact with each other through newsletters, conferences, and, increasingly, through the Internet.

The main strategy of Healthy Cities at the local community level is to create specific projects intended to act as catalysts for changes in policy. Commitment by political leadership to promoting the ideal qualities of a healthy city is an essential element of the strategy. These qualities include a clean, safe physical environment, a stable and sustainable ecosystem, a supportive community, public participation in decision making, and the meeting of basic needs such as food, shelter, and employment, among others (WHO, 1992). Healthy Cities emphasizes that it is the process of developing these qualities that defines a healthy city rather than some objective measure of health status.

Typical projects are managed by multisectoral committees with a membership composed of interested citizens and people and organizations that have the potential to influence the community's health (political and business sectors, education, housing, social services, environmental protection, and urban planning, among others). Such committees are linked to the political system of the city. Local project offices provide technical support, and almost all resources for activities are provided by the cities themselves. Research is conducted as an element of many Healthy Cities projects, and an international network of Healthy Cities researchers has been established.

There is substantial variety from city to city in the kinds of projects undertaken, the level and kind of technical support provided by project offices, and the composition and management style of the project committees. An interim review of Healthy Cities in Europe found that annual budgets for administering city projects ranged from nothing to XEC 618,000 (USD 700,000 in 1993 dollars). One third of the cities had a coordinator who worked less than half-time, but the mode was 1.5 full-time equivalent (FTE), and one well-staffed city had 4.5 FTE (Curtice, 1993).

Differences in resources and staffing aside, all participating cities are encouraged to go through a common process of planning and action that begins with finding, recruiting, and educating key decision makers about the Healthy Cities approach. A core group then assesses community needs and assets, develops a project plan, and secures political support for the project. A project coordinator is identified, and the project is put into action (Draper et al., 1993).

Projects in many of the cities have focused on one of three arenas for action: groups with special needs such as children, women, and the elderly; issues such as diseases and the physical environment; or geographical areas such as economically deprived neighborhoods and road accident problem areas. Many illustrative case studies have been published, and the interested reader is directed to several collections of case studies for details (Ashton, 1992; Davies & Kelly, 1993; Draper et al., 1993).

Healthy Cities: Research

Unlike the CVD prevention projects already discussed, Healthy Cities was not conceived primarily as a research project. It has no common protocol or measures of processes and outcomes but is rather "high risk and pluralistic" (Curtice, 1993, p. 36). Furthermore, Healthy Cities has no firm time frame for implementation and completion. As a self-feeding, self-sustaining political process, its size, course, and directions were unplanned and its incredible expansion was unanticipated.

Europe. Nevertheless, elements of Healthy Cities have been researched. The WHO European Regional Office coordinated an early review covering the first 2 to 3 years of the project, based on questionnaire and interview data obtained from the 25 cities in the European network at the time (Tsouros & Draper, 1993). At that early point in the project, the cities had made good progress in developing structures and processes but were still in the early stages of implementing programs.

A general finding was that the interval between obtaining political support for a project and the achievement of changes in a city's policies and programs was longer than had been anticipated. The main conclusion of the review was that success in implementation was related to eight factors, or qualities, that varied from city to city. These qualities were strong political support, effective leadership, broad community control, high visibility, adequate resources, sound administration, intersectoral cooperation, and strong accountability (Curtice, 1993; Tsouros & Draper, 1993). Assessment of a city project for these qualities can be used to assist faltering cities to regain momentum and to assist new cities in the project to success.

The review also revealed six priority areas where research was needed (Tsouros & Draper, 1993): (a) the health status of the economically and socially disadvantaged and its influence on the quality of their lives; (b) the health impact of poor housing, inadequate food, and limited education (among other basic needs) at the city and neighborhood levels; (c) the impact of urban policy on health; (d) constraints on intersectoral cooperation; (e) barriers to community participation and structures and processes to overcome them; and (f) strategies for better application of research in the health and social policy arena.

An expanded review was undertaken 5 years into the program that included 35 project cities worldwide. It was intended to help Healthy Cities learn more about how programs developed and provide insight to improve the second 5-year phase of the project (Draper et al., 1993). It found, predictably, that some cities had done a great deal and others had done very little, and that degree of political commitment and resources were important determinants of activity level. Most city projects were very general, encompassing a range of work and not specific to just one focused problem. The most successful projects had steering committees representing both the community and key agencies and were closely linked to the political system. They had specialized groups for management and technical support, the roles and responsibilities of committees and working groups were defined clearly, and projects were staffed at the level of a full-time coordinator or more.

In many cities, the establishment of a Healthy Cities program was in itself the main project activity, and the most important function of the project in the early stage was communication, stimulating new activities for health promotion carried out primarily by others in the community (Draper et al., 1993). A number of cities have, in addition, mounted projects with foci on research, policy analysis, planning, consultation, training, and neighborhood development.

Only 15 of the 35 cities in the review had begun or completed the preparation of comprehensive city health plans, which in an important sense is the main objective of the Healthy Cities approach to health promotion (Draper et al., 1993). In a more intensive study of this issue conducted in 10 cities in the Netherlands and the United Kingdom, it was observed that most city projects had managed to influence public policy to some degree, but few had had so clear an impact that new policy could be attributed mainly to the Healthy Cities project (Goumans & Springett, 1997).

The Netherlands. In addition to programmatic reviews, various Healthy Cities initiatives in Europe have been conducted in an action research frame, made possible by university-community partnerships. As part of Amsterdam's Health in City Boroughs project, for example, researchers at the University of Utrecht focused on the problem of how research on health needs could be a tool to promote health action, as opposed to research resulting in no action (ten Dam, 1996). The case study that was used to explore this problem was an intervention project in North Amsterdam, one of 18 city boroughs, aimed at improving the health of Turkish and Moroccan immigrants concentrated in the area.

The methodology combined qualitative and quantitative approaches. Epidemiological data were supplemented by information obtained in interviews with workers in the health care sector. The interviews served a dual purpose: to gather information on how the health services viewed the immigrants' health situation and to sensitize health care workers to the special circumstances of the immigrants living in the community. In-depth interviews were conducted with Turkish and Moroccan people to develop a better appreciation of the health cultures of these immigrants. The information obtained from all sources was discussed in several rounds of conferences aimed at developing consensus among the professional and lay conferees about priorities for action.

This work led to a proposal for a neighborhood health information center that would provide walk-in consultation, courses, and self-help groups, as well as written information on health topics. A steering committee including representatives of the health, social, and education sectors and the public took responsibility for implementing the plan. The Borough Council provided financial support. The collaboration grew, attracting new members from the alcohol and drug use arena and from a foundation for the welfare of the elderly.

Much of interest was learned in this project (ten Dam, 1996). The needs assessment process was effective in stimulating action. At the same time, the methodology was complex, very time consuming, and might be difficult to replicate in a community with scarce resources. As the project developed, health professionals tended more and more to become intermediaries for the immigrants. As the agencies involved were mostly health related, it was difficult to address determinants of health residing outside health services, such as cultural and economic considerations. The project continues as of this writing, and the complete story has yet to be told. But even at this stage, it is a clear demonstration of the feasibility of the participatory research approach in the Healthy Cities context.

Australia. At the time of the worldwide review of the 35 cities (already discussed), 650 cities in total were associated with the Healthy Cities movement in Europe alone, judged by the reviewers as the most significant indicator of progress (Draper et al., 1993). In other parts of the world, the European model of Healthy Cities was being adapted to local conditions. In Australia, for example, it was used as a mechanism for a cooperative approach to health planning and urban administration (Harris & Wills, 1997). Three pilot projects and a national secretariat were established, located in and mostly funded by the health sector. Australian projects have dealt with a wide range of issues including air pollution, water quality, housing, and safer environments for women, but their involvement in planning and work with local governments has been limited. Healthy Cities has not had as much penetration in Australia as in Europe, with but 17 of 800-odd municipalities having been designated as Healthy Cities projects after 5 years of the program (Harris & Wills, 1997).

It has been suggested that, on the Australian scene at least, Healthy Cities would have been better welcomed had it been more explicit about its social and environmental goals, as this might have helped relieve concern about the project's seeming lack of focus (Harris & Wills, 1997). Lack of uniformity thus appears to have been both a strength and a weakness in Healthy Cities in Australia and, perhaps, in other parts of the world. Lacking a sharp focus, Healthy Cities is open to suspicion ("What is this really about?"), but, lacking focus, the project can easily evolve in different forms in different places (Harris & Wills, 1997).

Canada. The European model also inspired action in North America, with rather different variants arising in Canada and the United States. In Canada, the birthplace of the Healthy Cities idea, the success of the project in Europe sparked renewed interest in the concept but with several twists (Hancock, 1993). Named Healthy Communities, to include explicitly the many small communities in Canada, the project was organized as a partnership of the Canadian Public Health Association (a nongovernmental organization), the Canadian Institute of Planners (the professional society of urban planners), and the Federation of Canadian Municipalities.

Most interestingly, the project was headquartered at the Canadian Institute of Planners, with a steering committee drawn from all three organizations, whose membership is dominated (purposefully) by the municipality sector (Hancock, 1993). The project is also distinct from the European model in that communities who wish to participate need not undergo a screening and selection process—it is open to any community that wants to join.

United States. Healthy Cities in the United States began in Indiana, with a grant from the W. K. Kellogg Foundation to fund collaboration between Indiana University, the Indiana Public Health Association, and six Indiana communities (Flynn, 1993; Flynn, Rider, & Ray, 1991). It was different from the European and Australian approaches in that it was begun explicitly as a partnership of researchers and community, set up to conduct action research to promote political action and social change.

The community development model used in Indiana assists people to examine critically the community in which they live and to increase their skill and involvement in solving community health problems (Flynn, 1993). Healthy Cities Indiana views community leadership development as a critical part of the process, similar to the European approach. It emphasizes placing health on the political agenda of the city, urges community leaders to consider the health effects of their decisions, views health as a shared responsibility in which the health sector plays a part, and promotes development of healthy public policy (Flynn, 1993).

Research in the project has addressed four areas of impact: leadership development and its dissemination, development of action programs, involvement of policy makers in public health, and policy change. A clear example of how the action research ideal has been put into operation in the Indiana model is its use of "effectiveness inventories" to provide information to Healthy Cities committees that enables the committees to make positive leadership changes and other alterations to develop more effective committees. The research effort also tracks policy changes that can be attributed to Healthy Cities. Documented examples of such changes include policies leading to curbside recycling of solid waste in two small cities and development of an environmental policy plan in one larger city (Flynn, 1993).

The Indiana project's research effort has also provided insight into ways the Healthy Cities process might be improved (Flynn, 1993). For example, committees with too many professional members experienced delays in action, in part because professionals usually do not carry out the work that committees decide on. There was a tendency, too, for health professionals and community leaders to control committee action, and if committees were not broad based enough, committees experienced some difficulty overcoming local vested interests. Healthy Cities in the United States has expanded beyond Indiana's borders, and in keeping with the diversity that characterizes the United States, the project has taken on different forms in different places.

This fluidity, in fact, has probably been crucial to the expansion of Healthy Cities, not just in the United States, but in Canada and Europe as well. At the same time, a practical consequence is that Healthy Cities, which is not one approach to health promotion through community development but many approaches, cannot be evaluated in the uniform way that has been possible with the disease prevention approach to health promotion at the communitywide level.

Knowledge Development in Healthy Cities

Davies and Kelly (1993) have pointed out that there is a natural tension between research and practice in Healthy Cities, partly because the project has not been based on an underlying academic tradition, partly because the research base for the Healthy Cities approach is in its infancy, and partly because the project's social-ecological-political processes are not particularly amenable to study using the biomedical research paradigm that many health researchers are trained in (pp. 1-13). Davies and Kelly call for an expansion of the frame for knowledge development in programs such as Healthy Cities, to include the biomedical approach but also use of stories, anecdotes, anthropological and journalistic reports, and qualitative, ethnographic, and action research methods. Science alone, they conclude, "cannot be used to solve such complex and multi-disciplinary problems as found in the health environment of cities" (p. 4).

Respecting Diversity

Communitywide health promotion is, self-evidently, a very broad arena. Some health promoters working in this arena view disease prevention through lifestyle modification as their key objective.

Others believe that health promotion's most important work is to influence political processes, thus stimulating improvements in the social, environmental, economic, and political conditions that are the "real" determinants of a community's health. Too frequently, in this writer's experience, proponents of various viewpoints are ignorant of, or seriously misunderstand, other perspectives.

Parochialism is exacerbated by the culture and language differences among the many countries where health promotion-related work is taking place, not to speak of widely differing academic traditions (biomedical and socioecological, for example) that cut across national boundaries. One result, at a practical level, is that practitioners and researchers working with health promotion in different parts of the world have not learned as much from each other's efforts as might be desirable.

At a more philosophical level, health promoters of all stripes have been faulted for failing to be introspective about the nature of health promotion practice and research and the biases and preconceptions they carry. Critics have pointed out a number of practical and conceptual dilemmas that follow from imprecision in the way important terms are defined and health promotion's relative lack of theoretical grounding (Lupton, 1995; Seedhouse, 1997).

Within academia, health promotion may become, but is not yet, a discipline. In the human and health services arenas, health promotion is, for many, an opportunistic arena of action with many guises. Program labels are often chosen based on political and funding considerations. A community-based tobacco control program, for example, might easily be labeled health promotion, or disease prevention, or health education, or primary prevention (or all of these!), with no real consideration given to the meanings of these labels.

Rather than viewing the situation with despair, the present state of health promotion at the communitywide level should be seen as an inevitable, early stage in its maturation process. By pointing to some of the meaningful lessons from two very diverse traditions in the community-based health promotion arena, as has been attempted here, it is hoped that this diversity will be recognized as a strength of health promotion, not a weakness. This chapter, with its illustration of, and plea for, diversity, also sets the stage for many of the case illustrations in both Part I and Part II of this book.

Finally, the reader will, of course, notice that no attempt has been made here to compare and contrast the two traditions in communitywide health promotion that have been discussed. For reasons that one hopes are obvious, that would be truly an apples-to-oranges comparison. Nevertheless, it is impossible to resist one such comparison. Despite all the differences—philosophical, scientific, practical, political—that distinguish these two streams of work, there does appear to be at least one common thread connecting the two. That is the application of community organization principles and processes in approaching communities: doing community analysis, working with communities, sustaining effort, and disseminating new knowledge. These subjects are taken up in detail, especially in Chapters 2, 3, 4, 5, and 7.

2

Social Change Theory

Applications to Community Health

BETI THOMPSON

SUSAN KINNE

The increasing focus on "community" in health promotion is due, at least in part, to growing recognition that behavior is greatly influenced by the environment in which people live. Proponents of community approaches to behavioral change recognize that local values, norms, and behavior patterns have a significant effect on shaping an individual's attitudes and behaviors (Abrams, Elder, Carleton, Lasater, & Artz, 1986; Carlaw, Mittelmark, Bracht, & Luepker, 1984; Farquhar et al., 1977; McAlister, Puska, Salonen, Tuomilehto, & Kosketa, 1982; Puska et al., 1985; Thompson, Lichtenstein, Wallack, & Pehacek, 1990-1991; Wallack & Wallerstein, 1986). This recognition has been paralleled by a call for new ways to achieve behavioral change. Rather than emphasizing change made by individuals, this "new" community approach argues that permanent, large-scale behavioral change is best achieved by changing the standards of acceptable behavior in a community; that is, by changing community norms about health-related behavior (Abrams et al., 1986; Carlaw et al., 1984; Farquhar, 1978; Farquhar, Maccoby, & Wood, 1985; Stunkard, Felix, Yopp, & Cohen, 1985; Syme & Alcalay, 1982; Thompson et al., 1990-1991; Wallack & Wallerstein, 1986).

Since publication of the 1970 World Health Organization (WHO) report on community initiatives, increasing attention has been paid to community organization as a means of achieving large-scale change in both primary prevention and treatment of chronic health problems (Blackburn, 1983; Carlaw et al., 1984; Elder et al., 1986; Farquhar, 1978; Green, 1986). The authors of the WHO report agreed that community organizations could change the community setting to support healthier lifestyles. That change would be translated to reductions in individuals' health risk behavior that would, in turn, lead to decreases in chronic disease morbidity and mortality.

The community organization approach to health promotion is based on the "principle of participation" (Abrams et al., 1994; Green, 1986; Green & McAlister, 1984; Thompson et al., 1990-1991; Wallack & Wallerstein, 1986), which asserts that large-scale behavioral change requires those people heavily affected by a problem to be involved in defining the problem, planning and instituting steps to resolve the problem, and establishing structures to ensure that the desired change is maintained (Florin & Wandersman, 1990; Goodman & Steckler, 1990; Green, 1986; Thompson et al., 1990-1991; Vandevelde, 1983; Wallack & Wallerstein, 1986). The "principle of ownership" is closely related to the principle of participation. *Ownership* means that local people must have a sense of responsibility for and control over programs promoting change so that they will continue to support them after the initial organizing effort (Bracht, Thompson, & Winner, 1996; Florin & Wandersman, 1990; Kahn, 1982; Kettner, Daley, & Nichols, 1985; Lichtenstein, Thompson, Nettekoven, & Corbett, 1996). Both principles follow from the same basic premise: Change is more likely to be successful and permanent when the people it affects are involved in initiating and promoting it.

In the last 20 years, a number of major health promotion initiatives have used a community approach to change behavior (Abrams et al., 1986; Carlaw et al., 1984; Cohen, Stunkard, & Felix, 1986; COMMIT Research Group, 1991; Elder et al., 1986; Farquhar et al., 1985; Fortmann, Taylor, Flora, & Jatulis, 1993; McAlister et al., 1982; Mittelmark et al., 1986; Puska et al., 1985; Tarlov et al., 1987). With few exceptions (e.g., COMMIT), most of these efforts addressed multiple risk factors related to cardiovascular disease, with goals of changing smoking, dietary, and screening behavior. All of them described themselves as "community projects" and used different community institutions, organizations, groups, and individuals in the delivery of the interventions. Most also emphasized public education through mass media, schools, and other organizations.

The majority of these projects recognized the need to change the social context of their communities, arguing that the environment has a significant influence on facilitating or inhibiting the adoption of new behaviors (Carlaw et al., 1984; COMMIT Research Group, 1991; Farquhar et al., 1977; Farquhar, Maccoby, & Wood, 1985; McAlister et al., 1982; Puska et al., 1985). Some researchers discussed the importance of changing community norms; documentation of such changes could be used as measures of the success of their projects. Community organizations were seen as means to achieve social context changes and normative changes.

Despite this emphasis on the community and community organization, in practice, the existing community projects paid little attention to norm and value change and seldom measured such change, relying instead on assessing individual change (Farquhar et al., 1985; Leventhal, Clearly, Safer, & Gutmann, 1980). In the area of smoking, for example, traditional approaches have been focused on changes in the individual (e.g., current smoker or not; long-term quitter or short-term quitter), with little or no attention given to the broad social context in which the individual acts. A great deal has been accomplished at the individual level. Smoking cessation programs have proliferated so that no smoker need look very far for help in quitting.

The Community Intervention Trial for Smoking Cessation (COMMIT) was one of the first to recognize that the smoker functions in a social context or social environment that contains many cues to continue the smoking habit (COMMIT Research Group, 1991; Thompson et al., 1990-1991). Some of the cues are easily identified (e.g., advertising of cigarette brands, addictive properties of cigarettes); others are more subtle (e.g., insurance or government subsidizing the costs associated with tobacco-related diseases). As ever more information emerges about the manipulation of the tobacco industry and its influences in a myriad of societal sectors, efforts for tobacco control have shifted from a focus on the individual smoker to a focus on public policy to change the social environment (ASSIST Program Guidelines, 1991).

The lack of empirical attention paid to changing community norms and values can be partially attributed to the lack of comprehensive theories explaining how such change occurs. Health promotion change programs tend to be primarily driven by "middle-range" theories that address the process of changing behavior among individuals or some component of the community (Elder et al., 1986; Farquhar et al., 1977; Green & McAlister, 1984; Maccoby & Alexander, 1980). There are, however, sound theoretical underpinnings that can be used to develop a more comprehensive conceptual framework for community change.

In this chapter, the process of change in the social context and in community norms is tied to a broad theoretical framework. The chapter is organized into the following parts: (a) the general principles of systems and communities, (b) general sociological perspectives of change, (c) the middle range of process theories concerned with changing specific components of the community, (d) a synthesis and application to community change, and (e) assessment of community change.

General Principles of Communities and Systems

For well over a hundred years, social scientists have been engaged in the systematic study of communities. From this work, at least two important principles can be identified. The first relates to definitions of community and the second applies a systems perspective to communities.

Community. Many definitions of community have been devised (Bell & Newby, 1971). The majority of definitions explain that a community is more than a mere aggregation of individuals; however, beyond that, communities may fall on a continuum from requiring little interaction among members (e.g., residents in an inner city) to regular, intimate contact (e.g., families). Warren (1958) provides a succinct definition that forms the basis for the one given here. Overall, communities can be defined as a group of people sharing values and institutions; specifically, some *social meaning* as well as some organizational structure must connect the individuals to the community. One community component included in the past was geographic proximity or locality; however, in the world of electronic communication and the ability to rapidly join meetings and conferences, it is not clear that locality is as important a factor as it once was. One important component of a community is that it has a sphere that provides a method for the *production, distribution, and consumption of goods and services*. This refers not only to durable goods, but also intangibles such as schools and churches. Communities also need a system of *socialization* to communicate their norms and values to new community members; typically, this is done through schools for children. For adults, socialization blends with *social control*. A variety of community components are needed to fulfil social control, including formal laws, rules within workplaces and other organizations, social ridicule, and other informal ways to keep individuals informed of the important aspects of a particular community. Another key component of community is that it must contain *interdependent social groups* that provide the basis for interpersonal relationships and mutual support.

This interdependence leads community members to help each other in times of trouble. Interdependencies can vary from very small units (e.g., families) to large formal agencies (e.g., the police department). An underlying principle of this definition is that communities form a whole greater than the assemblage of individuals within them (Bell & Newby, 1971).

Systems. The second principle can be found in a systems view of the world: Simply, communities can be viewed as systems. An inherent assumption of views of general social structure and change is that societal structures are systems that are long lasting, functionally interdependent, and relatively stable (Ashby, 1958; Boulding, 1978; von Bertalanffy, 1962). The system is based on some degree of cooperation and consensus on societal goals, norms, and values. The system, however, is not a simple aggregation of its component parts; rather, it is a unique structure that includes all the parts and the relations that connect them. The system provides the context for all activities, including making choices about behaviors. Thinking of a community from a systems perspective allows a better understanding of the interconnections of the various community levels, sectors, relationships, and members.

The community system includes individuals, subsystems, and the interrelationships among the subsystems. At least a century of sociological and anthropological work has identified important subsystems of any community system. These are the political sector, economic sector, health sector, education sector, communication sector, religious sector, recreational sector, and social welfare sector. In addition, community organization studies have identified two additional sectors as being important for achieving changes in the community system. These include voluntary and civic groups, such as health-related agencies, political action groups, and other grassroots groups, and other groups that may be specific to particular communities. The subsystems listed are neither mutually inclusive nor exclusive; they are intended to provide an example of some of the sectors considered important in a community. A schematic of the community system and its various parts and relationships is presented in Figure 2.1.

The view of the community as a system provides some insights into community organization for change. From a systems perspective, change in one sector usually implies that adjustments or responses will eventually occur in other parts of the system. Thus it is clear that community change may begin at any level of the community. Change that begins with one sector, however, may take a long time to affect the entire system. In addition, many factors may interrupt or divert the change effort. Typical examples of such factors include changes in community agendas, changes in resources available, and changes in organizations that have taken a leadership role in addressing a specific issue.

From a community organization perspective, the target of change is generally the entire system—the community itself. Making changes at the system level will maximize the rapid dissemination of those changes throughout the various sectors of the system. For such change to occur, new rules for appropriate behavior must become a part of the total system of community. From this perspective, it is not enough to change only a sector or part of the community, although changes in the sectors or subsystems, especially the political and economic spheres, may contribute to overall system change.

Because change is the goal of most community intervention studies, it is important to understand how and why such change is likely to occur. Many theories have presented views on this topic, and these are reviewed in the next section.

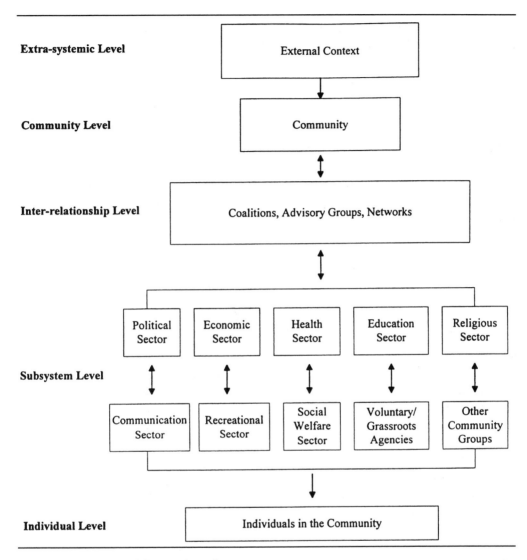

Figure 2.1. Schematic of Community as System

General Sociological Perspectives of Change

Social change is regarded as "the significant alteration of social structures (that is, patterns of social action and integration), including consequences and manifestations of such structures embodied in norms (rules of conduct), values, and cultural products and symbols" (Moore, 1963, p. 34). Social change is generally regarded as change in large social structures, and such change is generally preceded or followed by changes in the normative structure of a system. Norms are the shared rules and expectations that govern everyday life (Robertson, 1977), and they produce the regularity of behavior that allows individuals to be part of a larger social group. Normative change takes place when a shift occurs in the rules that govern behavior. The shift applies not only to specific individuals but to expectations governing behavior for the entire system or subsystem within which it occurs.

Two major perspectives have been used to explain social change: functionalist and conflict views. In general, functionalist theories emphasize patterns and processes that maintain a system (Cancian, 1960; Hempel, 1959; Nisbet, 1973; Parsons, 1951); conflict theories see imbalance as a constant part of any system, resulting in ongoing adjustments (Dahrendorf, 1959; Domhoff, 1969; Frank, 1967; Mills, 1959). Proponents of the two perspectives hold correspondingly different views on social change.

Proponents of the functionalist view see social change as a gradual, adaptive process oriented toward system reform. Systems, from this perspective, are based on cooperation and consensus, especially in the areas of societal goals, norms, and values (Robertson, 1977). Social norms are viewed as the links that help hold the system together. Social change occurs when parts of the system break down and are no longer able to contribute to system maintenance, or when external or environmental changes overwhelm the system. Social norms change along with the system to provide new rules of conduct to help maintain the reformed system. An example of this can be seen in emerging norms surrounding tobacco use. Technical changes—recognition of the dangers of smoking and of inhaling secondhand smoke—are leading to restrictions in public smoking. The tobacco industry says it is developing "safer" cigarettes. As the secular trend to protect individuals against the dangers of tobacco accelerates, smokers find it is no longer appropriate to light up in all settings, tobacco manufacturers are called to task for their contribution to the tobacco problem, and new rules for smoking must be developed.

Social change theories based on the conflict view see social change as occurring when one of several interests in a system gains ascendancy (Domhoff, 1969). Social norms, as in the functionalist view, help maintain a system, but in a coercive, rather than consensual, sense. Those who control important parts of a system, especially the economic and political sectors, establish the social norms, and attempts to change norms are likely to be met with resistance by them. Again, the norms regarding tobacco use can be used to illustrate this perspective. The tobacco industry, with its significant economic resources and strong lobby, maintains advertising privileges and secrecy as to the content of tobacco products. In addition, the industry has managed to define smoking as an individual choice or problem—a social norm upheld until recently in civil cases against tobacco companies (e.g., the 1988 New Jersey case, *Cipollone v. Liggett et al.*). A change in social norms, from this perspective, will result when an opposing interest group, such as antitobacco advocates, is able to exert more influence over the parts of the system now controlled by the tobacco industry. Recent examples include the view that nicotine is an addictive substance, class-action suits that have been decided in favor of entire groups of individuals (e.g., flight attendants), and the efforts of the tobacco industry to establish a settlement with states that have been responsible for paying for smokers' tobacco-related illnesses. Between 1990 and the present, a very different set of norms regarding smoking has prevailed than was previously held.

In these two system-level or "macro" theories, different aspects of society are seen as the causes of change. Both views confirm that impetus for change originates both within and outside of the system, although functionalists usually emphasize extrasystemic factors to which the system must adjust, and conflict theorists look for internal inequities and inadequacies as explanations for change. Although functionalist and conflict perspectives provide a framework for describing systems, their parts, their interactions, and change, they do not specifically address the processes of change. To understand those processes, an examination of specific theories is required.

Middle-Range and Process Theories of Change

The general principles of the social change theorists are supplemented with more than half a century of work in communities. From that background, as well as some other contexts, a set of process theories that addresses community change has been developed. These include theories at the individual, organizational, community, and environmental levels.

INDIVIDUAL-LEVEL CHANGE THEORIES

Individual-level theories of change are plentiful in the health promotion literature. Individual health is, after all, the ultimate goal of many health promotion activities. Stemming largely from the field of psychology, theories that focus on individual change may be categorized into two basic classes: (a) those that focus on intrapersonal characteristics of the individual, and (b) those that emphasize interpersonal factors as a basis for decision making.

Intrapersonal-level theories are those that examine individual characteristics, motivation, and other unique factors that may enhance or detract from behavior change. These internal constituents are considered of primary importance in many decisions about health. Theories that fall into this category often provide diagrams of how various components contribute to health behavior. The health belief model (HBM), for example, assumes that the likelihood of an action is shaped by one's perception of his or her own susceptibility to the disease and the perceived severity of the disease, which together form the individual's perception of the threat of the disease. Perceived threat, however, can be modified by many factors, including sociodemographic factors (age, gender) and knowledge, as well as "cues to action," which include education, symptoms, and information about the disease or how to overcome it. The final decision about whether to change behavior is further determined by an individual's perceived benefits (versus perceived barriers) to change (Rosenstock, 1974; Rosenstock, Strecher, & Becker, 1988; Strecher & Rosenstock, 1997).

An entire series of intrapersonal theories is organized around a view that behavior is rational and determined by attitudes and beliefs. Again, individual behavior is based largely on internal perceptions that have been formed as a response to beliefs of what causes disease and whether or not those causes can be overcome. The best-known theory in this area is the Theory of Reasoned Action (TRA) (Ajzen & Fishbein, 1980; Fishbein, 1990). This view assumes that the single best predictor of whether a person will change behavior is *behavioral intention*. That intention is shaped by attitudes toward that behavior and perceptions of how others will view the behavior (called *subjective norm*) (Ajzen & Fishbein, 1980). Recent updates to the TRA include the expanded theory of reasoned action (Montaño & Taplin, 1991) and the theory of planned behavior (Ajzen, 1991). Each of those theories adds additional factors to explain some aspect of behavior: For example, the expanded theory of reasoned action added affect and facilitating conditions as critical components of behavior change (Montaño & Taplin, 1991; Montaño, Thompson, Taylor, & Mahloch, 1997), and the theory of planned behavior added perceived behavioral control as a significant predictor of behavior change (Ajzen, 1991). Many more theories emphasizing the intrapersonal determinants of behavior can be found, but the foregoing are probably the best examples of the emphasis on the individual's internal processes as the primary element of change.

The other main class of individual theories of change includes the interpersonal theories. In these theories, the emphasis is on the importance of the relationships individuals have with friends, families, and others in their environment. It is thought that these relationships will influence behavior change. Social learning theory (SLT) is perhaps the best known of the interpersonal theories.

Explaining the interplay of knowledge, attitudes, and behavior has always been a challenge for psychology. The social learning approach recognizes that simple cognitive acquaintance with new material is not sufficient to motivate individual change (Bandura, 1969). Social norms and values, often implicit in this approach's description of behavioral acquisition, set limits on what will be considered and how easily it will be accepted. This suggests that a change in norms, however accomplished, will contribute to a change in people's learning and in their eventual behaviors.

Bandura's social learning approach is one of the most familiar models of change used in the health field (see, e.g., Bandura, 1969; Elder et al., 1986). In brief, the individual is regarded as a self-determining organism who acts on and reacts to environmental stimuli and acquires new ideas and behaviors by modeling them on focal others. In practice, this type of change is promoted by exposure to these role models. This is accomplished by mass media that increase access to the new ideas and behaviors, by use of prominent people as change initiators, and by exploitation of existing social networks that maximize interpersonal contact (Bandura, 1969; Lasater et al., 1984). Creation of social networks or linkages among people ("networking") is another ancillary technique to improve the likelihood that a target individual will learn and adopt a new behavior from those around him or her.

A theoretical framework that cuts across many of the individual-level theories of change is the Transtheoretical Model (TTM), also known as the "stages of change" model. The essence of the model is that behavior change occurs through a number of somewhat sequential stages: (a) *precontemplation*, during which an individual has no intention of changing a behavior; (b) *contemplation*, during which individuals intend to make some changes within the next 6 months or less; (c) *preparation*, during which change is anticipated within the next 30 days; (d) *action*, during which changes are being made but are not sufficient to be considered a permanent health behavior change (e.g., smoking cessation for 1 day; exercise for 1 day); (e) *maintenance*, during which behavior change is continued over time and relapses, if any, become increasingly rare and of short duration; and (f) *termination*, during which the behavior change is permanent and there are no inducements to return to the old behavior (DiClemente & Prochaska, 1982; Prochaska & DiClemente, 1983; Prochaska, DiClemente, & Norcross, 1992). Change from one stage to the next, or back to an earlier stage, occurs through processes or activities that are needed to move to the next stage. Sample processes are finding out about a behavior (consciousness raising), understanding the negative health impact of a behavior (environmental reevaluation), removing reminders of the unhealthy behavior (stimulus control), and substituting healthier behaviors for the unhealthy ones (counterconditioning) (Prochaska & DiClemente, 1983; Prochaska, Norcross, & DiClemente, 1994). The TTM has been applied to many behaviors, and some researchers have included other theoretical perspectives as part of the change model (Thompson, Shannon, Beresford, Jacobson, & Ewings, 1995).

Theories of collective action, especially those that emphasize rational choice, also can be applied to individual-level change; they presume that rational calculation of individual interest is the basis for decisions to participate in or abstain from particular activities (Heath, 1976; Olson, 1965). Critics of this approach argue that the theory is not an explanation of behavior but a description of behavior based in exchange theories; that is, people usually act as if they were rational. Proponents reply that what is important is the accuracy of the prediction, not the realism of its assumptions about behavior. This suggests that changes in the incentive structures of an individual will alter his or her behavior. For some behaviors, this approach works well (Becker, 1977). People may be convinced to perform well in their jobs in return for higher pay. In other situations, the role of the incentive structure is less clear. People may continue to drink or smoke even though there are penalties or deterrents attached to those behaviors.

ORGANIZATIONAL-LEVEL CHANGE THEORIES

Clearly, the individual need not be the only source of system change. The systems perspective recognizes that changes in subsystems and their interrelationships can also influence the system. The subsystems of a community consist primarily of organizations and individuals within them who work toward a common goal. The political sector, for example, may include organizations that promote certain political positions, groups responsible for governance, and individuals who hold political office. Organizational theories are useful in understanding how key organizations within a system can contribute to systemwide change.

Organizations and institutions can be altered in ways that are distinct from change in their membership (Grusky & Miller, 1981; Scott, 1981). Organizations are systems in themselves and espouse their own norms and values; thus they are also capable of change (Ermann & Lundman, 1978; Zey-Ferrell & Aiken, 1981). As Rogers and Shoemaker (1971) make clear, organizations learn and change through a process of diffusion. Networks between organizations facilitate diffusion of ideas and practices. The leadership structure of an organization may support change in response to changing external or internal conditions, and this is likely to have an effect on individuals within the organization. Good examples can be found in the area of organizational deviance, where individuals within an organization may find themselves following "company orders" that contradict social norms (Ermann & Lundman, 1978; Grusky & Miller, 1981). The classic heavy electrical equipment antitrust cases of the 1960s revealed that company officials repeatedly and willfully violated antitrust laws, yet these officials, to a person, stated that they were only following company policy (Geis, 1978).

The extensive literature on organizational change details the many forms such change may take. Organizational change may result from collective action or social movements (Gusfield, 1962; Olson, 1965; Zey-Ferrell & Aiken, 1981). Many occupational health and safety regulations have their roots in such movements. External changes may lead to shifts in the internal power of groups; new leadership may then pursue its own interests within the organization. A good example is the appointment of Surgeon General C. Everett Koop, whose agenda for his organization included an emphasis on the dangers of tobacco use.

Organizational development (OD) theories are based on Lewin's (1935) work and that of others who fostered changes in the environment of workers rather than merely controlling the workers. As with other organizational-level theories, this theory is primarily concerned with solving organizational problems, increasing productivity, and fostering good management-employee relations (Porras & Robertson, 1987). In applications to health promotion, OD theory focuses on the organizational environment. Recent studies have included management and employees in developing and institutionalizing health promotion activities at the worksite (Abrams et al., 1994). Similarly, personnel from schools have become involved in planning and implementing health programs (Goodman, Tenney, Smith, & Steckler, 1992).

Interorganizational linkages may also change the structure of organizations. A variation of the social network approach has been applied to this kind of change (Cook, 1977). In this view, mobilization and involvement of key community organizations will provide the impetus for total community participation in a change program (Cohen, Stunkard, & Felix, 1986). The key organizations network with each other and, in a manner congruent with diffusion theory, the "change" spreads throughout the community. For many proponents of this view, community change is simply the aggregated activities of the organizations.

COMMUNITY-LEVEL CHANGE THEORIES

At the level of the community as a whole, some theoretical approaches for change have been designed. The most familiar is probably that formulated by Rothman (Rothman, 1979, 1996). Rothman (1979) describes three general ways to intervene in a community for the purpose of community change: locality development, social planning, and social action. Locality development emphasizes the participation of community residents in identifying and solving a problem. Community capacity for change is high, consensus about a problem and solution is possible, and the change agent is seen as an enabler or facilitator of change. The social planning approach is based on rational planning and problem solving. Planners, often external to the community, may identify particular problems and implement activities to solve the problems. Community members are often consumers of the process. The social action approach is usually based in conflict and requires a dramatic shift in power, usually in favor of disadvantaged groups.

In recognition that the three models have significant overlap, recent work in this area has focused on how the three approaches may work together. An updated model, for example, identifies the types of organizational models that are likely to lead to specific intermixed forms of community intervention (Rothman, 1996). This new approach provides some valuable strategies for knowing which of the models to mix in specific situations. Rothman provides an example where human service professionals need to establish a halfway home for adolescents in a specific neighborhood. Although such an activity falls into the "social planning" approach, there is much to be gained by what Rothman calls "symbolic participation" in accepting the halfway home (Rothman, 1996).

A key component of each of Rothman's three views is that community members are involved in community change. This involvement has, however, a number of possibilities (from simple acquiescence of the community members to total decision making). A number of recent studies suggests that community members take on aspects of capacity building (Jackson et al., 1994), community development (Labonte, 1993), and community "regeneration" (McKnight, 1987). All of those views are oriented to returning more power and control to the community. They are still considered "community organization" strategies, but a preferable label appears to be *community empowerment* (Florin & Wandersman, 1990). There is even a question as to whether external researchers should go into communities and "create" a change agenda, as that is seen as a role for the community (Freire, 1970). Others, however, have argued that some accommodation can be made (Thompson, Corbett, Bracht, & Pehacek, 1993; Thompson, Lichtenstein, et al., 1990-1991).

The social work tradition of community organization, combined with anthropological insight about cultural differences, has given rise to the field of community development (van Willigen, 1976). (This is not to be confused with what Rothman and others refer to as community development, which is a broader field of social and economic improvement and has much more in common with what Rothman refers to as "locality development.") In the anthropological version of community development, local participation may be encouraged, but the emphasis is on economic development that is harmonious with the native culture. The outcome is community change, but the concern is less with process than with efficient achievement of this economic aim. Its normative consequences are of secondary interest. Nevertheless, this approach has some useful ideas for community change efforts; for example, providing resources to the community can help expedite the achievement of desired individual behavior changes.

Another view of community change relies heavily on organizational relationships. In the health field, such relations are fostered when diverse organizations within a community come together to form coalitions to address problems (Koh, 1996; Marty, Nenno, Hefelfinger, & Bacon-Pituch, 1996; Snyder, 1997). Numerous large-scale health promotion projects (e.g., the American Stop Smoking Intervention Study [ASSIST], Robert Wood Johnson Smokeless States awardees) are currently using coalition approaches to influence community change. Coalitions are generally thought to be alliances of various organizations within a community. The alliance agrees to work together for common goals. Previously, we saw how some theorists viewed community change as the aggregated activities of organizations. In the coalition version of this view, proponents identify organizations and their linkages as "the community" (ASSIST Program Guidelines, 1991; Elder et al., 1986). A sizable literature details how this organizational network may be conceptualized and measured (Burt & Minor, 1983; Goodman, Burdine, Meehan, & McLeroy, 1993; Mulford, 1984). Because of its sophisticated methodological development, it can provide useful indicators of change in community structure and function. For example, changes in decision making, power, and influence can be tracked to ascertain what groups are having the primary impact on a community (Galaskiewicz, 1979). Altman et al. (1991) examined the obstacles to and future goals of 10 communities that had coalition-driven health programs. Many obstacles were identified by the coalition members, and it was not always clear that the goals could be attained.

Community organization has taken on a somewhat different perspective internationally. In 1986, the World Health Organization (WHO) initiated the "Healthy Cities" movement. The partnership in healthy cities includes both governmental and nongovernmental sectors and focuses on policy change and the reduction of health-related inequities (Tsouros, 1995). This contrasts with the stance in the United States, where the focus on public policy change is relatively new.

ENVIRONMENTAL-LEVEL CHANGE THEORIES

When we speak of community change, we rely implicitly on our ability to distinguish "community" from its environment. This ability may be analytical rather than practical, but it does allow us to think about external sources of community change. Environmental-level theories of social change are important because external stimuli can influence the system. Secular trends in national norms, for example, may have an impact on the community system, just as at the organizational level, exogenous shifts can change the balance of power at the community level.

Economic theories of supply and demand provide one framework for describing this process of adjustment (Becker, 1977). Entire communities, for example, have declined because industries have moved out of town when demand for their products decreased or when cheaper workers could be found elsewhere. In many cases this kind of change requires the community to make significant adjustments to maintain the components of its system; that is, schools, jobs, services, and so on. Social movements can also affect the larger environment, thus constraining or changing the options open to particular systems (Gusfield, 1962; Troyer & Markle, 1983). The civil rights movement of the 1960s required new formal and informal norms about relationships among people in a variety of settings. There may also be policy changes at a higher level—state laws or regulations, for instance—that affect a community in a completely exogenous manner. The American Disabilities Act, workplace smoking restrictions, and increases in taxes are all good examples of such externally imposed constraints on behavior.

In summary, a number of theories at various levels have been used to explain how communities or other systems can change. Most of the views suggest strategies that could be used as part of an effort for community change. In the next section, these views are synthesized and applied to a specific issue.

Synthesis and Application to Community Change

The general principles and discrete theories discussed above have been applied in a variety of settings and have achieved some level of empirical support. They have not yet been integrated into a larger theoretical framework of community change; nevertheless, we can use them to present a synthesis that draws from theories at each of the levels discussed earlier. Schematically, this integrated approach is represented in Figure 2.2. Communities can be considered systems. General sociological theories can help explain how the system is held together as a whole, and the middle-range or process theories can be used to explain how change occurs within the components of the system.

As depicted, the system is stable (functionalist view), with most of the system components (e.g., individuals and subsystems) in consensus on societal goals (e.g., community development and planning), norms, and values. Within the system, however, there are vested interests that act to preserve the status quo, and collective action or social movements may arise to counter those vested interests (conflict view). The system also interacts with the environment. External stimuli, in the form of laws and policies, secular trends, critical events, or technology may influence norms and values within the system. The external stimuli may lead to social movements or collective actions to change community behaviors. Change within the community may be planned either internally or externally. External forces often use social planning or locality development theories to orchestrate change. "Partnership" arrangements between internal and external resources are common.

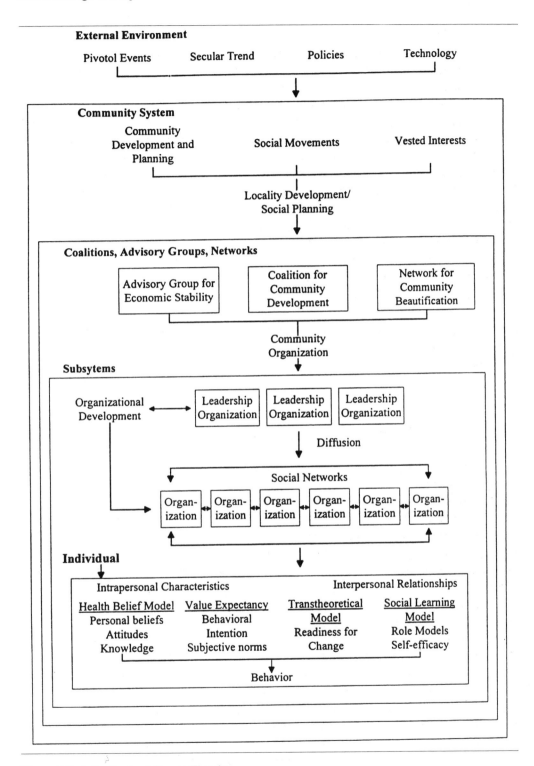

Figure 2.2. A Synthesis of Change Theories

Community organization strategies may be used to mobilize a community around a problem. This may result in a number of advisory boards, coalitions, or networks emerging to address specific issues (e.g., economic stability). Whether falling into locality development, social planning, or social action, various activities may occur at the community level to promote change.

At the subsystem level, various important organizations work together to achieve change in the community. Social network theory and interorganizational theory explain how such connections are initiated and sustained. As various groups become involved, the change is diffused to other groups in the community. Theories that explain this process include diffusion theory, organizational development, and interorganizational relationships. Some organizations may take on leadership roles and thus become more important than other subsystems as change agents. Especially critical are the political and economic subsystems; they are frequently able to move a change in norms from the organizational level to the community level.

Individuals, because they interact with the subsystems, are subjected to changing norms and practices at the subsystem level. New norms may be reinforced by role models who make the appropriate behavior change. Social learning theory explains how individual change may occur in response to such role models. New information may have an effect on an individual's decisions; similarly, the expectations of others may influence an individual's behavior. Eventually, because of organizational change and change in subsystems and their interrelationships, new norms prevail, and widespread individual change is likely to occur. This synthesis provides a theoretical explanation for activities that have been used singly or in varying combinations in community projects. It can be applied to a variety of community projects attempting to achieve community change.

ILLUSTRATION

As an illustration (see Figure 2.3), consider the case of the Community Intervention Trial for Smoking Cessation (COMMIT) (COMMIT Research Group, 1991, 1995). This was an example of an externally initiated community project targeting smoking cessation and, to some extent, prevention. On the environmental level, the project itself might have been regarded as an external stimulus to the community. Another external stimulus was the growing secular trend to treat smoking as an activity that affects the entire public, not merely the smoker who practices the habit (system theory). As a result, some collective actions (employee agitation for smoke-free work areas) and small social movements (Doctors Ought to Care, Americans for Nonsmokers' Rights) addressed the issue of smoking. In addition, changes in smoking policy at the national, state, and local levels may have had some impact on the local community.

At the community level, project investigators worked with community organizations to "sell the project" to the community by uniting organizations and individuals in defining smoking as an important issue. As key influential groups began to support the project, there remained the possibility of vested interests opposed to the project (e.g., Smokers' Rights groups, local tobacco industry representatives). By providing some resources (community development, economic theory) and establishing a base of expertise from which the community could draw (community development), the investigators sought to integrate themselves with community leaders and groups (interorganizational approach). Through the social networking process, subsystems within the community system linked together through a Community Board and Task Forces to address the

The FoCaS Project

Improving Breast and Cervical Cancer Screening Among Low-Income Women

ELECTRA D. PASKETT

CATHY M. TATUM

RALPH D'AGOSTINO JR.

JULIA RUSHING

RAMON VELEZ

Breast and cervical cancer account for one third of new cancer cases and 18% of cancer deaths among women in the United States (Landis, Murray, Bolden, & Wingo, 1998). The impact of these cancers, as for most cancers, is greater among older, low-income, and minority women (Miller et al., 1993). These women tend to underuse screening tests (Cervical Cancer Control, 1991; National Cancer Institute Breast Cancer Screening Consortium, 1990; Weinberger et al., 1991) resulting in more late-stage cancers and poorer survival rates (Mandelblatt, Andrews, Kerner, Zauber, & Burnetta, 1991; Wells & Horn, 1992). Factors related to lower screening rates and higher breast cancer mortality rates in this population include: failure of physicians to recommend screening (Gemson, Elinson, & Messeri, 1988; Weinberger et al., 1991), limited access and referral to preventive and therapeutic services (Kirkman-Liff & Kronenfeld, 1992; Whitman et al., 1991), and negative beliefs about the disease process and the medical community (Lerman, Rimer, Trock, Balshem, & Engstrom, 1990; Zapka, Stoddard, Costanza, & Greene, 1989).

In an effort to address breast and cervical cancer screening in these women, the National Cancer Institute initiated a research program titled "Public Health Approaches to Breast and

Cervical Cancer Screening," with a focus on addressing barriers and developing clinic-based and community-focused interventions to improve the use of these screening exams (National Cancer Institute Cancer Screening Consortium for Underserved Women, 1995). Three projects were funded in 1990 (Minnesota, Rhode Island and Texas) and an additional three projects were funded in 1992 (Wisconsin, West Virginia, and North Carolina). Each project was unique in its setting and types of clinic-based and community outreach interventions used; however, all projects focused on improving breast and cervical cancer screening among underserved women 40 years old and older. This paper reports the results of the North Carolina project, which used multiple behavioral theories and had the goal of improving beliefs, attitudes, and screening behaviors of women 40 and older who resided in low-income housing communities.

Methods

Overview

The objectives of the Forsyth County Cancer Screening Project (FoCaS) were to reduce the burden of breast and cervical cancer by improving knowledge, attitudes, and participation in breast and cervical cancer screening and to identify barriers to screening faced by women and health care providers. Secondary objectives were to improve compliance with follow-up recommendations for abnormal findings from mammography and Pap smears. The project was conducted in low-income housing communities located in two cities and was implemented in four phases over a 4-year period. In Phase 1, surveys among providers from health facilities that serve the population and surveys among women in the housing communities were conducted to assess breast and cervical cancer screening knowledge, attitudes, and practices. A community advisory board (CAB) from the intervention city was also formed in the first year of the project. Members of the CAB either lived in the communities or represented organizations that served the residents of the community, such as the Winston-Salem Housing Authority and the city government. The role of the CAB was to provide input on all aspects of the study, from how to gain access to the community to reviewing intervention and survey materials.

In the second phase, the in-reach (community- and health center-based) and out-reach (community-based) interventions for screening and follow-up of abnormalities were implemented in the housing communities in the intervention city. Phase 3 involved a follow-up survey of women; Phase 4 included the transfer of successful interventions to the comparison city. A mixed cohort and cross-sectional design was used to evaluate the success of the intervention (Koepsell et al., 1991). Independent cross-sectional surveys, conducted before and after the intervention, were used to assess community trends in mammography and Pap smear screening over time. The cohort was formed by randomly selecting half of the women who had participated in the baseline survey. These women were interviewed again in Year 4 to assess the effects of the intervention on screening rates over time on individual women. In this case illustration, only data from the cross-sectional surveys will be presented. The FoCaS project also included a consortium of local community agencies, including a community health center, a medical school located in the region, Wake Forest University School of Medicine (WFUSM), the health departments and public housing authorities in both cities, a historically African American state university (Winston-Salem State University), community organizations that focus on cancer (e.g., American Cancer Society and Cancer Services), and the Winston-Salem Urban League.

Setting

The FoCaS project was conducted in Winston-Salem and Greensboro, North Carolina. The population of interest consisted of women, predominantly African American, residing in low-income housing communities, 40 years old and older. In Winston-Salem, nine housing communities with 908 women formed the intervention group. In Greensboro, 18 housing communities with 1,024 women formed the comparison group. The baseline characteristics of this population have been reported elsewhere (National Cancer Institute Cancer Screening Consortium for Underserved Women, 1995).

The clinic-based strategies to improve screening rates were focused in a community health center in Winston-Salem, Reynolds Health Center (RHC), which provides multispecialty clinics in pediatrics, adult medicine, and obstetrics and gynecology for low-income residents of the county and in-house mammography as well as other medical care on a sliding fee scale basis. In Greensboro, the comparison clinics included a free community clinic, the Urban Ministries Clinic, and the outpatient clinic of Moses Cone Hospital. A total of 174 physicians (including residents) practicing at these health care facilities participated in this project. The demographic and practice patterns in terms of breast and cervical cancer screening of these physicians are described elsewhere (Paskett, McMahon, et al., 1998).

Surveys

The baseline and follow-up surveys of knowledge, attitudes, barriers, and use of breast and cervical cancer screening among women in the population were conducted by interviewers. The baseline survey began in November 1992, was completed in March 1993, and achieved a response rate of 82% for the intervention city and 73% for the comparison city. A total of 124 surveys were completed in Winston-Salem and 120 in Greensboro. For the follow-up survey, only women who resided in the communities during the intervention period were eligible for sampling. This survey began in October 1995, concluded in June 1996, and achieved a response rate of 84.5% in the intervention city and 68% in the comparison city. A total of 163 surveys were completed in Winston-Salem and 138 in Greensboro. Analyses of the race and age of women who refused to complete a survey did not find any differences compared to women who participated in the survey.

INTERVENTION DESIGN

To develop effective interventions, results from the baseline women's survey, the health care provider survey, additional focus groups, and input from the CAB were used. These sources provided information on barriers, attitudes, current breast and cervical cancer screening practices, and optimum strategies for delivering health education messages. The development of the multicomponent clinic-based and community-based interventions is described in detail elsewhere (Paskett, McMahon, et al., 1998; Tatum, Wilson, Dignan, Paskett, & Velez, 1997).

Theoretical Framework

The theoretical framework for the community-based interventions included the PRE-CEDE/PROCEED model for planning (Green & Kreluter, 1991); the health belief model (Bandura, 1977; Becker, 1974; Glanz & Rimer, 1995; Rosenstock, Strecher, & Becker, 1988) and the transtheoretical model (Prochaska et al., 1994) for identifying and addressing barriers; social learning theory (Bandura, 1977; Rosenstock et al., 1988) in terms of using lay health educators to deliver education messages; and the PEN-3 (person, extended family, neighborhood—third revision) model (Airhihenbuwa, 1993) to incorporate cultural appropriateness and sensitivity in program development. Four of these models have been described in the preceding chapter; however, the last model, the PEN-3 model, is unique to this study.

The PEN-3 model consists of three dimensions of health beliefs and behavior that are dynamically interrelated and interdependent (health education, educational diagnosis of health behaviors, and cultural sensitivity and cultural appropriateness of health behaviors). This model is one that addresses cultural sensitivity and cultural appropriateness in program development for health education of African Americans (Airhihenbuwa, 1993). For example, the FoCaS logo (see Figure CI2.1), used women of both African-American and Caucasian ethnicity and younger and older ages to convey a sense of identity with the women in the housing communities.

Implementation of Interventions

Analyses of information gathered for the PRECEDE model indicated that women had poor attitudes and knowledge about screening and faced barriers in terms of access to services (e.g., Where do I get a mammogram?). Few women had positive reinforcement from others to get screened. For the PROCEED portion of the model, it was decided that intervention activities needed to inform women about the need for screening and where to get screened, and others needed to be involved—to obtain reinforcement for getting screening exams. These principles then guided the development and implementation of the intervention activities. In addition, the PEN-3 model provided the framework for incorporating culturally appropriate graphics, role models, and channels (e.g., African American newspapers) for the delivery of intervention messages.

Interventions implemented in the housing communities during the 2-year intervention period included Women's Fest, a free party held in the community that included food, educational classes, cholesterol, blood pressure and diabetes screening, prizes, and information booths; a church program that included a ministers' luncheon and Taking Care of Our Sisters (a lay educator program for female church members); educational brochures especially designed to address identified barriers such as where to get a mammogram; mass media techniques such as bus ads and newspaper and radio ads on African American media; monthly classes in each housing community conducted by a lay health educator; birthday cards with the FoCaS logo; targeted mailings and door knob hangers with invitations to events; and one-on-one educational sessions in women's homes.

Clinic-focused interventions implemented at RHC were designed to address provider, system, and patient barriers to conducting breast and cervical cancer screening. These interventions included in-service and primary care conference training for providers on issues including

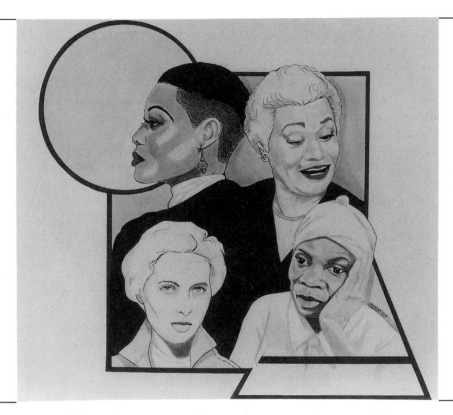

Figure CI2.1. The FoCaS Logo

clinical breast exam (CBE) proficiency, cultural sensitivity, and techniques to integrate preven-tion in primary care; visual prompts in the exam rooms (e.g., "Have you screened today?"); educational games (e.g., "Find the Lump Game") to teach CBE techniques; an abnormal test protocol which included alert stickers, a referral process for managing the care of women with abnormal test results, and a tracking system; poster and literature distribution in the waiting rooms; and one-on-one counseling sessions and personalized letters for follow-up testing for women who had abnormal test results.

ANALYSIS

Descriptive statistics were calculated for demographic and health care characteristics by time (baseline and follow-up). These statistics were compared using t tests, and unadjusted chi-square tests and logistic regression models were used. The outcome for these models was compliance with mammography and Pap smear screening guidelines, defined as follows. For mammography, women between 40 and 49 years of age were within guidelines if they had received a mammogram within the last 2 years, and women 50 and older were within guidelines if they had received a mammogram within the last year. For cervical cancer screening, women who had received a Pap smear within the last 3 years were defined as in compliance with guidelines. In these analyses, we first fit a model with main effects for time (pre- and post-), city (intervention and comparison), and a Time × City interaction. For this model, the odds ratio corresponding to the Time × City interaction was of greatest interest, as it represented to what extent the Pap smear (or mammogram) usage rate increased in the intervention city relative to the comparison city over the duration of the study. In addition to these unadjusted models, we also used the logistic regression models, including race, age, and education as covariates. Using the same modeling techniques, we examined whether the proportion of women reporting that someone had encouraged them to get screened was different over time in each of the two cities and whether the change over time was different in the two cities.

To assess the effectiveness of the intervention, we examined the women in the cross-sectional follow-up survey in the intervention city to determine whether a higher proportion of women who attended a FoCaS class were regular screeners compared to those who did not attend a class. To assess this, we calculated odds ratios based on 2 × 2 tables of women who were regular screeners (yes or no) by FoCaS class attendance (yes or no) for both Pap smear and mammogram. To determine whether there were changes in stage of readiness to obtain a mammogram for women at baseline compared to follow-up, women were grouped into appropriate stages (as defined by Skinner, Strecher, & Hospers, 1994) and a four-degrees-of-freedom chi-square test was used.

Results

CHARACTERISTICS OF THE SAMPLE

Demographic and health care characteristics of the women in the cross-sectional sample are shown in Table CI2.1 by city and time period. On average, women were between 65 and 68 years old. About 60% of the women in both cities at both time periods were age 65 or older. The majority of women were African American, with significantly more African American women surveyed in the intervention city at both time periods (78% vs. 65%, $p = 0.02$ at baseline; 92% vs. 64%, $p = .001$ at follow-up); this, however, represents the racial distribution in the housing communities of the two cities. The majority of women had health insurance, and women were evenly distributed among the three education levels (less than 8th grade, 9th to 11th grade, and high school graduate). As the study was conducted in low-income housing communities, income was not assessed; however, all women were in similar economic levels, and few women in either community under age 65 were employed (15% to 30%). Fewer than 20% of the women were currently married, and the majority had been pregnant (85%). About 30% of the women were current smokers, and 80% to 85% had had a regular checkup in the last 12 months. No other differences in sample characteristics were noted between cities over time.

SCREENING RATES

Pap smear use rates for women in the cross-sectional samples are shown in Table CI2.2. The proportion of women who received a Pap smear within the last 3 years increased in the

TABLE CI2.1 Demographics and Health Care Characteristics of the Sample by City and Survey

| | Baseline Survey (N = 244) | | | | Follow-Up Survey (N = 301) | | | |
| | Intervention (n = 124) | | Comparison (n = 120) | | Intervention (n = 163) | | Comparison (n = 138) | |
Variable	n	Percentage	n	Percentage	n	Percentage	n	Percentage
Age								
40 to 64	54	44	53	44	59	36	53	40
≥ 65	70	56	67	56	104	64	85	60
Education								
< 8th grade	54	44	44	37	56	34	42	32
9th to 11th grade	40	32	39	33	59	36	44	33
High school or above	30	24	37	31	48	29	47	35
Employed (and < 65 years old)	12	22	15	28	15	25	14	30
No health insurance	19	15	17	14	17	10	8	7
Smoking status								
Never	62	50	56	47	80	49	54	46
Ever	22	18	30	25	40	24	33	28
Current	40	32	34	28	44	27	31	26
Marital status								
Married	22	18	24	20	23	14	20	15
Ever married	88	72	86	72	115	70	98	73
Never married	13	11	10	8	27	16	16	12
Race[a]								
African American	97	78	78	65	151	92	86	64
Had regular checkups	98	80	96	79	134	82	165	85
Parous	106	85	102	85	136	82	101	85

a. For intervention versus comparison city for baseline survey, p = .02; for intervention versus comparison city for follow-up survey, p = .001.

TABLE CI2.2 Pap Smear and Mammography Use Over Time

	Community					
	Intervention		Comparison			
Sample	Pre	Post	Pre	Post	Unadjusted, OR (95% CI)	Adjusted,[a] OR (95% CI)
Percentage with Pap smear in last 3 years	73 (n = 122)	87 (n = 167)	67 (n = 122)	60 (n = 116)	3.3 (1.5, 7.3)	3.2 (1.4, 7.2)
Difference pre to post	+14		−7			
Percentage with regular mammograms[b]	31 (n = 125)	56 (n = 165)	33 (n = 123)	40 (n = 134)	2.0 (1.0, 4.2)	1.9 (0.9, 4.0)
Difference pre to post	+25		+7			

NOTE: OR = odds ratio; CI = confidence interval.

a. Adjusted for race, age, and education.

b. Regular is defined as in the last 2 years for women 40 to 49 years old and last year for women 50 years old or older.

TABLE CI2.3 Effect of Intervention on Stages of Change for Mammography[a]

	Stage (%)[b]				
	Precontemplation	Contemplation	Action	Maintenance	Relapse
Time					
Baseline	17.9	34.1	26.0	3.3	18.7
Follow-up	9.7	24.2	11.5	40.0	14.5

a. Adapted from Skinner et al. (1994).
b. $p = .001$ (chi-square test).

intervention city from 73% to 87%. The proportion of women reporting a Pap smear in the last 3 years in the comparison city decreased over time, from 67% to 60%. Thus, the Pap smear usage rate increased by 14 percentage points in the intervention city and decreased by 7 percentage points in the comparison city, for an overall increase of 21 percentage points in the intervention city relative to the comparison city. The unadjusted odds of increasing Pap smear use was 3.3 times higher in the intervention than in the comparison city (95% confidence interval [CI] 1.5-7.3). After adjustment for race, age, and education, the odds ratio was not significantly changed.

Mammography use rates are also shown in Table CI2.2. In the intervention city, 31% of women reported having had a mammogram within guidelines at baseline, and 56% reported having had one within guidelines at follow-up. The percentage of women reporting that they had had a mammogram within guidelines also increased in the comparison city, from 33% to 40%. The overall percentage point increase in the intervention city was 18 for mammography use relative to the comparison city. Although not statistically significant, women in the intervention city appeared to be 1.9 times more likely to have increased their mammography use after adjustment for age, race, and education (95% CI 0.9-4.0) compared to women in the comparison community.

ASSESSMENT OF INTERVENTION EFFECTS

As described earlier, the theoretical framework of the study was based on multiple models of behavior change. Several outcome measures were assessed to examine the effects of the intervention in relation to these models. Women were classified into appropriate stages in the Transtheoretical Stages of Change Model as described by Skinner et al. (1994) at baseline and at the follow-up survey. As shown in Table CI2.3, at baseline most women in the intervention city (34%) fell into the contemplation stage; at follow-up, most women (40%) were in maintenance ($p = .001$).

Barrier, belief and knowledge scales did not change appreciably over time (data not shown); however, certain items within these scales did change. Of interest are variables related to encouragement from others to receive a screening test, as this could be reflected in the lay health educator intervention. At baseline, 59% of women in the intervention city and 39% of women in the comparison city reported that someone had encouraged them to get a mammo-

TABLE CI2.4 Intervention Effectiveness, Percentage Regular Screeners[a]

	Attended a FoCaS Class			
Screening Test	Yes	No	OR	p Value
Pap smear	90.3	84.2	1.74	0.25
Mammogram	65.3	48.4	2.01	0.03

a. *Regular* is defined as in the last 2 years for women 40 to 49 years old and within the past year for women 50 years old or older; for Pap smear screening, *regular* is defined as having had one in the last 3 years.

gram. At follow-up, 83% of women in the intervention city and 44% of women in the comparison city indicated someone had encouraged them to get a mammogram. This percentage significantly increased in the intervention city ($p = .001$) but not in the comparison city. For Pap smear use, the proportion of women reporting that someone encouraged them to get a Pap smear increased in the intervention city (79% to 89%, $p = .017$). This proportion decreased in the comparison city over time (67% to 46%, $p = .001$). For both screening tests, the change in the intervention city over time was greater than that in the comparison city ($p < .01$).

Among women who resided in the intervention city, further analyses were conducted to examine the effectiveness of FoCaS intervention strategies. Overall, 66% of women had seen or attended at least one FoCaS intervention activity: 43% of the women attended at least one FoCaS education class, 28% had attended at least one of the three annual Women's Fests, 20% recalled seeing a FoCaS ad in the newspaper, 17% recalled hearing a radio ad, and 12% recalled seeing a FoCaS notice in a church bulletin. When regular use was examined by participation in FoCaS activities, effects of the intervention were noted. Table CI2.4 shows that women who attended a FoCaS education class were 74% times more likely to have had a Pap smear in the last 3 years than those who had not ($p = 0.25$). A stronger effect was found for regular mammography use (odds ratio [OR] = 2.01, $p = 0.03$).

Discussion

The goal of this study was to examine the effect of an intervention program which focused on clinic in-reach and community outreach techniques on improving rates of breast and cervical cancer screening among women 40 years old and older who resided in low-income housing communities. Multiple behavioral theories were used to design interventions for women. Cross-sectional data indicated an increase in both mammography and Pap smear screening among women in the intervention city. Examination of process evaluation data from the intervention city indicated that women who reported attending FoCaS educational classes were more likely to have received a mammogram within age-specific guidelines than those who did not attend a class. In addition, data indicate that women in the intervention city shifted from contemplation to maintenance over the study period. Lastly, there was an increase in the number of women in the intervention city who stated that someone encouraged them to receive both Pap smear and mammography screening.

Several limitations need to be kept in mind when interpreting these data. This study used only two cities and thus does not constitute a formal community trial. The study design did not provide all of the assurances of internal validity expected in a formal community trial; therefore the results cannot be used to estimate true intervention effects or actual screening rates over time. The fact that the unit of randomization, cities, was different from the unit of analysis, individuals, may have artificially decreased variance estimates and thereby increased the likelihood of finding a significant result (Kish, 1965; Murray, Hannan, & Baker, 1996). Randomization by housing unit was not an option because women in each unit in the intervention city received medical care at RHC, where clinic-based interventions were delivered. In addition, the use of more cities was limited by resources. Self-reports of screening were used; however, validation of self-reports of screening conducted on baseline data indicated good agreement for mammography self-reports (77% agreement) and fair agreement for Pap smear use (67% agreement) (Paskett, Tatum, et al., 1996).

The baseline and follow-up surveys were conducted within 3 years of each other for the majority of women. Thus, using a window of 3 years as a definition of compliance with Pap smear screening guidelines could overinflate the estimate of the intervention. This overestimate still does not account for the fact that the proportion of women in the comparison city who received regular screening decreased over time. To be included in the follow-up survey, women must have resided in the cities for the entire intervention period; thus, the rates of screening are not a true measure of screening rates in the cities but are relevant only for comparisons of changes in rates as presented. Although the strengths of the results are reduced by the study design features, the results do add more evidence to the possible acceptance of community interventions, especially those that use multiple strategies and multiple behavioral theories (Flynn et al., 1997).

Previous community studies focusing on increasing mammography and/or Pap smear use have also faced methodological difficulties. Of the 19 representative reports of community-based programs conducted to date, 8 included no control group as part of the evaluation design, 6 selected intervention and control communities and sampled women within each of the communities, and 5 sampled individuals within one or more communities or worksites and randomized them in some fashion (not always simple random assignment) to intervention and control conditions. Although many of the studies that employed no control group reported interesting intervention programs and positive results (Forsyth, Fulton, Lane, Burg, & Krishna, 1992; Gregorio, Kegeles, Parker, & Benn, 1990; Gresham, Molgaard, Elder, & Robin, 1988; Mayer et al., 1992; Saurez, Nichols, & Brady, 1993; Vogel, Peters, & Evans, 1992; Wilkes, Schoenfeld, Rursch, & Mettlin, 1988; Zapka, Harris, et al., 1993), deficiencies in the research designs do not allow generalization. The largest intervention effect for a community-based study was reported by Rimer et al. (1992): An intervention based on the Health Belief Model and Social Learning theory produced an effect of 33 percentage points.

The final goal of the FoCaS project was to disseminate intervention components within the comparison community and to continue the intervention efforts in the intervention community. This was, ideally, to be done through members of the consortium (e.g., the American Cancer Society, the Urban League, health departments); however, this goal was not accomplished. Future studies desiring implementation of successful components of community interventions by communities should review the principles and strategies outlined in Chapter 7 of this book.

The in-reach efforts, on the other hand, were continued at RHC. Thus, barriers to achieving long-lasting results from this study existed apart from the residents themselves. Other barriers that were encountered within these low-income communities included (a) concern for nonhealth issues (e.g., family responsibilities, work, safety) that reduced attendance at classes, (b) challenges to accessing individual women in larger communities, and (c) younger women being less receptive to health-related messages.

Future studies directed at similar populations may choose different approaches to avoid these barriers. One-on-one interventions might be more effective in reaching more women in low-income communities; however, the costs of this strategy may be prohibitive. A well-respected community spokesperson or representative could also encourage participation of residents better than study staff. This type of representative should be included in a study team. Lastly, limiting the number of channels in which the intervention is delivered (e.g., clinic-based or classes) may also be a better way to deliver information to low-income populations. Only by bringing such theory-based interventions to communities can true reductions in cancer mortality be achieved.

3

Assessing Community Needs, Resources, and Readiness

Building on Strengths

CHRIS RISSEL

NEIL BRACHT

Assessing the Community

Community analysis is the process of assessing and defining needs, possible barriers and opportunities, and resources involved in initiating community health action programs. This process is variously referred to in the literature as "community diagnosis," "community needs assessment," "health education planning," and "mapping." Analysis is a critical first step not only in shaping the design of project interventions but also in adapting implementation plans to unique community characteristics. It should define community strengths as well as potential problem areas. The product of community analysis is a dynamic community profile, blending quantitative health and illness statistics and demographic indicators with information on political and sociocultural factors. The profile includes a community's image of itself and its goals; its past history and recent civic changes; and its current resources, readiness, and capacity for health promotion activities. A review of previous (if any) community analyses and needs assessments is also important.

The process of completing a comprehensive analysis of the community can also provide a unique opportunity for citizen involvement in a community health project. In genuinely empowering and participatory health projects, analysis is not done *on* the community but *with* the community. Through involvement in the study process, citizens and organizations can develop awareness and "ownership" of the program and build commitment to local action. Studies of communities can rarely be completed if local citizens do not cooperate. The level of interest in a new project can be an early indicator of community readiness.

Many communities may already have conducted some form of community analysis or general needs assessment. Typically, these broad community analyses do not provide all the planning information needed for a specific project. Original data will need to be collected. New projects can therefore be seen to contribute to the broad understanding of a community. Sustainability of programs (see Chapter 7) is more likely if these programs build on existing efforts. Also, focused needs assessments can be an efficient approach to collecting relevant and timely information for program planning and engaging those people most likely to be interested in or affected by an innovative program.

In addition to its planning function, the process of conducting a community analysis is intended to lead to citizen activation and participation in a designated sustainable health intervention. In this chapter, we begin with a brief discussion on the meaning of community and then review the traditions and approaches that have influenced current community assessment and diagnostic models. This is followed by the presentation of methods for data collection, including suggestions for special studies to increase information about selected social groups in a community.

What Is Community?

In beginning a community analysis, one of the first questions asked is, What is a community? How is it defined? No single definition or concept of community serves all fields of investigation or professional intervention. Community has multiple meanings and has been studied from varying perspectives by sociologists, geographers, medical specialists, anthropologists, urbanologists, and social workers. However, as early as 1955 and after studying 94 definitions of community, Hillery (1955) found that 73% of definitions agreed that "social interaction, area, and a common tie or ties" (p. 118) were commonly found features of a community. Some define community as a psychological bond or relationship that unites individuals in a common goal or experience. Others use the term in the geographic or physical sense, as a space with political or economic boundaries. Yet space alone does not tell us all we need to know about community membership. The Internet and "virtual" communities can make physical, geographic boundaries obsolete.

Many characteristics of community structure and interaction have been identified in the writings of sociologists, including such useful concepts as community complexity, horizontal and vertical linkage among institutions, centralization of authority, regional autonomy, community identification, and social integration of the population. Theoretical underpinnings for this chapter rely principally on Warren's classic (1969) social systems view of the community, which focuses assessment on four important features—space or boundaries, social institutions, social interaction, and social control—and Chavis and Wandersman's (1990) view that communities can be identified by arbitrary geographical boundaries, by their social relationships, or through the exercise of collective political power. Sometimes these dimensions overlap, such as in isolated rural towns. For other communities, only one dimension may be present, such as in the case of a national coalition representing state-based grassroots organizations lobbying government for a single issue. The type of problem or intervention being planned and how community is defined will determine the nature of analysis required (see Chapter 2, pp. 31-32, for additional discussion).

In any analysis of a community, the geographical boundaries (or their absence) must be specified and should approximate the view held by most local residents or community members. Often, government health agencies have responsibilities for populations living or working in arbitrary geographical areas. Once boundaries are determined, an assessment of social institutions (education, health, recreation, business and labor, religious, communications and media, government, and so on) is undertaken to understand which organizations currently take responsibility for providing programs and services. Service directories may well list services provided, but a more thorough assessment also allows for the estimation of the possibilities for coordinating communitywide programs of health action. Social interaction patterns should also be studied for what they can reveal about community cleavages (for example, discriminatory practices), coalitions and influence networks, and sources of social support for individuals and groups (Heaney & Israel, 1997; House, Umberson, & Landis, 1988). An examination of social control mechanisms and norms is also useful. Social control is a function of many community institutions (church, school, police, and so on) and is based on values, norms, and customs. Any ethical concerns raised about a proposed community health intervention should be noted. How political power or the collective power of community members is used should be understood, as should local regulations and enforcement policies (e.g., concerning the sale of cigarettes to minors). Interviews with a variety of organizational and political representatives or key informants can provide most of this kind of assessment information.

Assessment Traditions

Before describing the various components of analysis, we briefly review the background of various assessment traditions. The terms *community analysis* and *community diagnosis* are used interchangeably in the literature, although analysis, strictly speaking, precedes diagnosis. The term *community diagnosis* surfaced in the 1950s (Morris, 1975) and was introduced to the health planning field in the mid-1960s. The content of community diagnosis was later reformulated by Bennett (1979). Green, Kreuter, Deeds, and Partridge's (1980) pioneering work "Health Education Planning: A diagnostic approach" added a broader social diagnostic framework to this applied discipline. They have extended this framework further to include environmental, policy, and legislative perspectives (Green & Kreuter, 1991). The World Health Organization (1982) has published a handbook for community health workers in the developing countries based on the community diagnosis concept. Haglund (1988) has written about community diagnosis within the Swedish context, and Hawe, Degeling, and Hall (1990) have described community needs assessment in the Australian context within a planning and evaluation framework. Other guides include Blum's (1981) *Planning for Health* and Dignan and Carr's (1986) *Program Planning for Health Education and Health Promotion*. Suggestions for how to approach community needs assessments can also be derived from major theories of personal and community behavior described in texts such as Glanz, Lewis, and Rimer's (1997).

Community analysis has evolved independently from two basic traditions that follow different paradigms that can broadly be termed the *health planning approach* and the *community development approach.* Some refer to them as "trickle down" or "bubble up" approaches. Elements from these two approaches can be found in assessment practice today, and the approaches can overlap.

The medical or health planning approach equates health with the absence of disease and health improvements with the application of medical science and technology to the community. The medical concept of community analysis in Sweden, for example, dates to the 18th century, when the Swedish Collegium Medicum requested that district medical officers record patterns of epidemic and endemic diseases each year and encouraged them to describe important factors that influenced these disease patterns in terms of demography, environmental health hazards, and living habits. This use of routinely collected public health data is a relatively common government approach to identifying health needs and priorities and could be seen as a minimal form of community analysis. In parts of Australia (Rissel, Winchester, Ward, & Sainsbury, 1995), routinely collected health data have been aggregated and presented according to national goals and targets frameworks. This allows ready identification of regional priorities. The health planning approach to community analysis can lack direct citizen involvement or consultation and tends to rely on diagnosis by experts.

The Canadian Lalonde report (Epp, 1986), using this approach, started a worldwide chain of national reports addressed to disease prevention. Other countries have similar approaches to national health goals and targets, such as reports of the Better Health Commission in Australia in 1986 and national goals and targets reported in the document *Better Health Outcomes for Australians* (Commonwealth Department of Human Services and Health, 1994). New Zealand has developed a strategic public health framework for improving health (Public Health Commission, 1994), as has England (Department of Health, 1992). In the United States, *Promoting Health and Preventing Disease: Objectives for the Nation* (U.S. Department of Health and Human Services, 1980), the surgeon general's report, *Healthy People 2000: National Health Promotion and Disease Prevention Objectives* (U.S. Department of Health and Human Services, 1991) reflect the health planning influence.

Priority areas for new health interventions are often determined by individual health providers or the community. Efforts to develop a planning process, however, usually follow a needs assessment model adapted from community social service planning. Health promotion planning is often isolated from other social service planning (especially in U.S. communities) and is often separate from major primary health care providers. This fragmentation in planning between health and social service areas is common and requires new approaches and solutions, by policy and legislative leaders, that are in the best interests of communities. For a further discussion of new partnership structures in health promotion planning and implementation, see Chapter 4.

Lack of coordination of services may never completely disappear, but often improvements can be made. For example, some states in Australia have created regional area health services that have a legislated responsibility to prevent ill health and to protect and promote the health of the people living and working in that area (New South Wales Department of Health, 1986). Each area has its own budget and is responsible for primary, secondary, and tertiary prevention and treatment services, from youth drop-in centers and community health staff to high-technology operating rooms. Services and programs can be matched to the needs of the community.

The community development approach views health in the broader context of social and economic improvement and views individual and community empowerment as vital to improvement in health status. Better health, in large part, is seen as the result of improvements in social and educational levels and involves improved quality of life as well as access to and control of medical and preventive programs and services. Community members are encouraged to take greater responsibility for and control of their own health. Community development emphasizes community cooperation. Advocates of this approach include Freire (1970), Nix (1978), Biddle and Biddle (1985), Bracht (1988), Rifkin (1988), and Minkler and Wallerstein (1997).

One example of the community development approach is the *A Su Salud* program, a community health program implemented in the low-income community of Eagle Pass, on the Mexican American border (Amezcua, McAlister, Ramirez, & Espinoza, 1990). A special feature of this program was its focus on interpersonal communication in cuing: providing feedback on and reinforcing the acquisition of health behaviors and attitudes that were promoted in mass media messages. An extensive network of "lay leaders" and volunteers participated in training programs to enhance communication within their social networks to promote and reinforce positive health behaviors. Volunteers served as role models in media campaigns or identified role models from their social networks across seven categories of sites: neighborhoods, business settings, government, social clubs, health care providers, education settings, and religious organizations.

The community development (or community organization) approach emphasizes direct citizen participation in the community analysis process and encourages a grassroots or "bottom-up" decision-making process rather than a "top-down" health-planning approach in which "experts" determine the community's health promotion agenda and new initiatives. Minkler and Wallerstein (1997) provide a good overview of this approach and present several U.S. examples. Other examples can be found in most countries in the world (Community Development in Health Project, 1988). More recently, coalitions of organizations have developed as major vehicles for collaboration (Butterfoss, Goodman, & Wandersman, 1993) and participation to achieve shared goals (ASSIST Project, NCI, United States, 1989-1998). The old adage that there is strength in numbers remains true, especially in policy and advocacy interventions (for example, smoking bans in public areas).

In an attempt to formalize the key processes of community organization, the U.S.-based COMMIT project required participating communities to engage in 12 specific activities to support its mobilization efforts (U.S. Department of Health and Human Services, 1995). Among these activities were the establishment of a community planning group, planning for a program office and staff recruitment, the first community board meeting, the creation of a task force member list and recruitment of members, writing of by-laws and organizational rules, development of a field site management plan, the preparation of a smoking control plan, annual action plans for each of the 4 years of the project, and the development of a transition plan for the postfunding period. To begin with, COMMIT researchers prepared a community profile for all communities in the trial using quantitative and qualitative information. Intervention communities also had more detailed assessment prepared to identify key stakeholders and relevant resources to avoid duplicating or replacing existing services. Communities where intervention staff were involved in this process found the community profile and analyses most useful. Thompson, Corbett, Bracht, and Pehacek (1993) have reported on the successful mobilization process of local community boards in the COMMIT project.

Health promotion planners following the community development paradigm view the community as both the context in which a health promotion program operates and the vehicle through which institutional changes in attitudes, practices, and policies can be effected. The information gathered for community analysis can facilitate partnerships among organizations, civic leaders, and groups that play an important intervention role as channels of program dissemination. Overlap of the two approaches can be found in programs such as PATCH (Planned Approach to Community Health) (Centers for Disease Control, 1992).

Components of Community Analysis

The purpose of community analysis for health promotion is to identify resources, problems, and opportunities and to set priorities for planning and developing an action program. The quantitative or descriptive aspect of this analysis has five components:

1. a demographic, social, and economic profile compiled from census or local economic development data resources;
2. a health and wellness outcomes profile (morbidity and mortality data);
3. a health risk profile (including behavioral, social, and environmental risks);
4. a survey of current health promotion policies, programs, and activity;
5. special studies of target groups, awareness levels, perceived needs, and organizational capacity.

Table 3.1 summarizes these components of community analysis and typical data sources and methods.

GENERAL COMMUNITY PROFILE (SOCIOECONOMIC)

First, geographic boundaries of the community must be defined in terms of political units or service areas. Data for this area of assessment include geographic, demographic, social, and economic factors. It is important to describe the community's population by age, sex, and ethnic heritage. Other social variables may include family structure, marital status, housing conditions, education levels, immigration, divorce rates, voting participation, crime rates, and available quality-of-life measures. Economic indicators may include employment, labor force characteristics, poverty and related welfare and social security beneficiary rates, general business conditions, and major economic developments. Communities with high unemployment or recent economic recession may have fewer resources and be less capable of achieving commitment to a "health focus" agenda.

HEALTH AND WELLNESS OUTCOMES PROFILE

The community's health and wellness profile reflects the distribution of illness and well-being in the community. This profile may consist of health indicators or single factors reflecting the health status of individuals or defined groups. National or state goals and targets identify key outcome indicators and usually include information such as age-specific death rates, proportional

TABLE 3.1 Summary of Community Analysis Components and Typical Data Sources

Analysis Question	Typical Data Sources
General community characteristics, structure, and history: What are the geographic features of this community? What are its unique concerns, social and health-related community agendas, and recent civic actions?	Wide range of social-economic sources: census information, economic development and social service data. Historical and other social indicators.
Health-wellness outcomes assessment: What are the levels of ill health and disability? Are there any indicators of wellness?	Epidemiological measures; past health or quality-of-life studies. Selective use of regional and national health data sources, including regional or state health departments.
Health risk profile: What are the behavioral, social, and environmental risks to the population and/or special subgroups?	Local health screening surveys or past risk factor studies from state or national sources and registries; behavioral risk factor telephone surveys.
Community health promotion survey: What programs, resources, skills, and provider groups already exist? What is the level of participation in these programs? What possibilities exist for collaboration? In what areas is there a need to develop or expand?	Current community inventories used to develop database through contacts with local informants: health departments, local medical clinics and hospitals, and nongovernment organizations.
Specialized studies: What special target groups or gatekeepers exist? Can they facilitate diffusion of program messages? What do these groups want to do? Who are the people who can help or hinder the project?	Systematic surveys or key informant interviews of special target groups, interviews with organization officials and reputed influential people or groups, leadership surveys.

mortality ratios, unnecessary deaths, potential years of life lost, and morbidity and mortality rates. The profile may contain composite measures summarizing data for defined target groups, such as young children, adolescents, or women. Comparisons of regional profiles with national or state targets (such as Healthy People 2000) may identify priority health issues or areas where wellness indicators are high or where health can be improved.

HEALTH RISK PROFILE

The health risk profile has three main components: behavioral risk, social risk, and environmental (physical, chemical, and biological) risk. Comprehensive assessment methods for each of these areas are available in the work of other authors (e.g., Green & Kreuter, 1991); we present here a brief summary of the salient features to be assessed.

The behavioral risk assessment includes dietary habits and use of drugs, alcohol, and tobacco, as well as patterns of physical activity. If previous studies are not available, studies of similar populations or in nearby areas may be applicable, or planners may choose to conduct their own surveys of community residents regarding health behaviors and perceptions of health problems and needs. Examples of service use by individuals or groups, self-care activities, and perceived needs can be included. Use of alternative health care programs (e.g., holistic medicine) can also be assessed.

Social indicators of risk are less commonly studied, but their utility may be of increasing importance. The stress of long-term unemployment, isolation, and/or poor education has been associated with poor health status. On the other hand, recent research suggests that positive health outcomes are related to social support mechanisms. New approaches to measuring social supports and networks are being reported in the literature. Gottlieb (1985) discusses variables that can be used to measure the source and strength of social networks. House et al. (1988) have reviewed the concepts of social support and their overall utility.

Environmental factors associated with health risks include the local quality of the physical environment, including water, soil, air, climate, and housing characteristics. Representatives of local and state environmental agencies should be interviewed to identify special problems in a particular community's environment.

COMMUNITY HEALTH PROMOTION PROGRAM SURVEY

Before planning or undertaking new health initiatives, it is important to have a complete description of current health promotion efforts in the community. One way to identify current programs in a community is to consult with key community informants on the status of community programming (Neuber, 1980). However, such efforts may be limited by the restricted experience and perspectives of these informants. As experts from the community, they have a better and more complete knowledge than do outsiders, but unless they have had to pull together a summary of current programs for some purpose, their knowledge is often incomplete and fragmented. A more comprehensive and objective procedure to describe health promotion programs is often needed.

An early effort to provide such a description of community health programs can be found in the Community Resource Inventory (CRI) procedure developed by the Pennsylvania Heart Health project (Cohen, Felix, & Yopp, 1986). The Minnesota Heart Health Program developed and expanded an assessment instrument (the Community Health Promotion Survey) that has the advantage of providing quantitative indicators of community health promotion activities, allowing evaluation over time of specific changes in the status of programming. (For a discussion of its use, see Weisbrod, Pirie, Bracht & Elstun, 1991). In assessing a community's health promotion program status, one wants to know where the community is concentrating its efforts and resources. An examination of program activities helps organizers judge the breadth of opportunities available to individuals in improving their health and highlights the areas of health where opportunity is low. A review of the type of strategies used by current health promotion programs (whether mainly educational or mainly attempting to change an environmental feature) may also suggest new approaches that could supplement existing ones (Rissel & Khavarpour, 1992). Examining the range of current programs and the extent and type of community participation they encourage can also help determine the need for additional programming.

SPECIALIZED COMMUNITY STUDIES

For planning purposes, there may be a need to secure additional information on the characteristics of selected social groups of the population. In the Minnesota Heart Health Program, for example, data on membership in community groups and associations were obtained (Carlaw, Mittelmark, Bracht, & Luepker, 1984). Church membership was high in all three intervention cities, ranging from 43% to 48%. Thus churches were considered as sites for community awareness and educational programs. Membership in sports and recreation groups ranged from 22% to 28%. About 50% of the groups that citizens belonged to provided some type of health information. Thus already-existing channels for health information dissemination were used.

Community groups may be the focus of health promotion programs, due to specifically identified needs. For example, there is considerable migration to Australia of people from non-English speaking countries. In some areas of Sydney, almost half of the population speaks a language other than English at home, with clustering of some language groups. After the Vietnam War, a significant population of Vietnamese people migrated to the southwest of Sydney. Anecdotal reports of high male smoking rates and worsening dietary habits suggested opportunities for health promotion, but little was known about this population. A survey of southwestern Sydney residents born in Vietnam was planned, but innovative methods of sampling needed to be developed and community support was needed. After extensive consultation with Vietnamese community groups and Vietnamese health workers, a community advisory committee was established to advise health department survey research and program implementation groups. This community advisory group was instrumental in identifying key cultural issues, in generating publicity prior to the survey, and in promoting community trust of the study. The survey identified very high rates of male smoking (Rissel & Russell, 1993) and was critical in successful advocacy efforts to fund a substantial community smoking cessation program that has since won prestigious multicultural marketing awards. This model of a community group as an advisory group was also applied successfully to a health education program for the Khmer community (Rissel, 1992).

STUDY OF COMMUNITY LEADERSHIP

Involvement of community leaders is essential to program success. The identification of influential persons and organizations should begin early in the community diagnosis process. Various approaches to studying community leadership and decision-making processes are detailed by Finnegan, Bracht, and Viswanath (1989). There are essentially four approaches to an analysis of influence and leadership: positional, reputational, decision-making, and community-reconnaissance forms of analysis. These alternative methods are based on different assumptions about community power structure and function. They were developed originally in formal sociological studies of communities located primarily in the United States, but they have their roots in ethnographic methods. Their current applicability to other societies has not been fully evaluated.

The "modified positional-reputational approach," as reported by Nix (1978), identifies different types of influential individuals or groups, based on leadership function (legitimizers, effectors, activators, and general public). The method also reveals community factions and key coordinating groups or centers of decision making whose involvement (or noninterference) may be critical for a health program's success.

Typically, a brief survey form is used to collect information. However, the size and scope of a leadership analysis should reflect the resources, time frame, and scope of the community needs analysis being conducted. More informal interviews may be sufficient in smaller studies. The energy of participants should not be expended unnecessarily for data collection if no one is left to conduct the intervention program! Basically, during personal interviews with leaders, the interviewer begins by describing the need or the proposed project and then answers any questions the interviewee might have about it. Next, the interviewer asks questions, including questions about other community leaders who might have interest in the subject or experience in other communitywide projects. The interviewee names other respected leaders and "doers" in the community. Examples of prior successful or unsuccessful community programs in health or other areas are also requested in these interviews. Finally, information is gathered on organizations that might be interested in or important to the success or failure of such a program.

These interviews are not only a tool for community analysis but a first step in the community organization process: They introduce the project or purpose of the study to the community. The reputational survey may result in 50 to 75 interviews, depending on the size and complexity of the community. The opinion leader survey (sometimes called a key informant survey) period usually takes several weeks. In one Minnesota community of about 35,000, leadership interviews were conducted with 30 informants who named the most influential persons in each community sector. The total number of times a leader was named served as a guide in making decisions about his or her influence and potential role on project task forces.

Leadership influence may operate differently in rural communities, where an individual's influence may extend beyond his or her own organizational boundaries. For further discussion, see Project Northland case illustration, p. 115, this volume. A guide to contacting key influential and institutional sectors of the community is provided in the Appendix to this chapter.

ASSESSING READINESS AND
CAPACITY FOR CHANGE

A critical area of qualitative diagnosis is the determination of readiness for and commitment to community change. If a key leadership study has been completed, information about the attitudes and expected level of participation of key community actors will have been obtained. A behavioral risk factor survey can pinpoint personal perceptions of needs and priorities among the general public. The extent to which a community and its leaders share a common vision of the future and have a record of past successful achievements is a good measure of how likely they are to become activated toward a new goal. McKnight (1988) has developed a methodology for mapping community capacity and assets.

Recent health demonstrations point to the importance of developing issue awareness before substantive community problems can be dealt with or changed. Unfortunately, many programs do not go beyond issue awareness. If community awareness is low, then careful marketing of health messages is a common approach to attempting to maximize community uptake and increase community readiness to participate in health promotion programs. Developing local awareness, then, is a prerequisite of goal setting and developing cooperative strategies for action.

Sometimes the inability to act on a problem occurs because the community lacks experience in using or developing resources in a concerted way. Conflicting agendas may not allow groups to prioritize communitywide problems or opportunities readily. Past leadership conflicts may impede groups' working together. Project organizers must recognize that participating organizations (e.g., voluntary health organizations) are unlikely to substitute new collaborative goals quickly for their own longstanding goals. Redefinition and/or modification of collaborative goals may be required, and this process has the best outcome when both groups approach it constructively. New research on sustainability of health promotion programs suggests that the closer a new program's objectives are to an organization's objectives, the more likely it is that the program will be adopted by the organization and the more likely the program is to continue (Bracht et al., 1994; Rissel, Finnegan, & Bracht, 1995).

Cottrell (1983) has developed a construct for viewing community competence. A competent community is one in which the various component parts have the following abilities:

1. They are able to collaborate effectively in identifying the problem and needs of the community.
2. They can achieve a working consensus on goals and priorities.
3. They are able to agree on ways and means to implement the agreed-upon goals.
4. They can collaborate effectively in the required actions.

These abilities represent, of course, an idealized model of community readiness. They serve as a general guide rather than a predictive set of absolute requirements. Examples of measurement of competent communities are rare (Eng & Parker, 1994). Interviews with key informants and organization officials can identify past achievements or conflicts and existing organizations or networks that will be needed. Focus group interviewing methods (see Krueger, 1988) can often be useful in this type of assessment. Locating sources of energy and enthusiasm is one goal in this analysis. Identifying target markets for programs is another. Project organizers need to examine their own objectives and energies as well. Does the sponsoring group have the experience to build a perception of credibility and trust in the community? Are project objectives consistent with the values of local community participation and ownership? Does the project maximize local resources? Are the project organizers prepared to be flexible in program design and/or implementation?

Summary

Successful implementation of community health promotion programs and interventions depends in large part on accurate analysis and understanding of many community and social factors. A community's history, including past collaboration among various sectors, is important, yet it is sometimes overlooked in the assessment process. Previous needs analyses can be helpful in providing much of this information and identifying gaps in knowledge. Specialized studies of target groups may be required. Community analysis is a comprehensive process used to assess health needs, organizational resources, leadership patterns, and potential for change. Results of these various analyses reveal not only a great deal about a community's health needs, but also the community's agenda and readiness in working toward program implementation and sustainable programs.

Key Community Sectors, Leaders, and Organizational Contacts

This summary list of key organizations and contacts can be useful in planning overall community assessment studies, especially the leadership survey, or in choosing target groups for highly specific needs assessments. Depending on the focus of the needs assessment, some organizations may not need to be approached.

Media
- local or citywide newspapers (publisher or editor, feature editors)
- radio stations (market area served and target audiences)
- TV stations (market area served and target audiences)
- billboard or other major advertisers

Health care providers
- health personnel (type and number)
- public and private health agencies, insurers, health maintenance organizations (HMOs)
- associations and societies for professional health care providers
- health department staff
- voluntary health agencies

Educational institutions
- schools or school districts serving the geographic area that defines your community
- school board members or principals
- number of students per grade per school

Government agencies
- key officers (e.g., county executive, mayor's office, city manager, political representatives, safety and planning officers)
- copies of health-related legislation and recent attempts to change health legislation

Economic and commercial organizations
- worksites and businesses from chamber of commerce reports
- estimated proportion of employees at large businesses
- unemployment rates
- key businesses with health concerns or programs

Labor organizations
- major trade unions

Religious groups
- general characteristics of main religions
- any interfaith council

Voluntary or private organizations (nongovernment)
- social, cultural, or sports groups
- service organizations (e.g., Lions, Rotary)
- community meeting places
- special communitywide events, sponsors, key activists

Community Capacity for a Breast Screening Program

The Lee County Experience (1991-1998)

JOHN K. WORDEN

BERTA M. GELLER

DONNA J. SABINA McVETY

ANNE L. DORWALDT

CATHERINE M. LLOYD

The goal of this project was to develop and evaluate a model community program to promote greater participation in breast cancer screening by women 40 years old and older, through public education and through education of medical professionals who provide screening. In 1990, when the study began, research indicated that less than half of women 40 and older received mammography screening at recommended intervals and that the performance of clinical breast examinations by physicians and breast self-examinations by each woman needed improvement to achieve full screening effectiveness (Worden, Mickey, et al., 1994). If this model community program was found to be successful in promoting greater screening participation over a 5-year test period, the program would be recommended for adoption in more communities.

Although this study began with a medical or health planning approach in which educational techniques found to be effective in previous research were to be applied in the community, it also incorporated a community development approach to implement the program when priorities from community leaders became clear during the community analysis process. To observe the impact of the community analysis process on the breast screening program, we will first review steps taken in conducting the community analysis, then describe the program elements that evolved from it, and finally examine the long-term durability of the program.

Community Analysis

ASSESSING COMMUNITY CHARACTERISTICS

The first step in community analysis was the selection of Lee County, Florida, as the community receiving both the planned intervention and evaluation surveys; a second site was selected as a comparison community receiving surveys only. Each study site was selected from a list of Florida metropolitan areas having a population of at least 75,000 women 40 and older. Communities of this size were required to provide sufficient statistical power to assess long-term breast cancer mortality benefits that could be achieved from greater participation in breast cancer screening.

Demographics of the two communities selected for the study were similar, with 1990 U.S. Census data indicating that 25% of the population in both communities were 65 years old or older (compared to only 12% in the United States as a whole), and both communities had patterns of income and education similar to each other. As melting pots of older Americans relocating in retirement, these communities reflected the profile of the U.S. population that can be expected in the next few decades. Each community also had well-defined populations of African American residents and equal amounts of lower income residents who were at increased risk of not getting screening.

Each of the two communities had well-dispersed hospital facilities that were both nonprofit and for profit, each had independent mammography facilities and active medical societies, and there was almost no managed care in either community in 1990. Each community had local county health departments and voluntary agencies, including the American Cancer Society. With adequate geographic separation, the communities provided an excellent comparison for evaluating a community-based intervention. Although initial meetings with community leaders were held as described below in both communities, Lee County, including the cities of Fort Myers and Cape Coral, was selected as the community receiving the intervention because its close proximity to a major airport provided ready access for out-of-state research staff traveling to support the program and its evaluation.

SURVEYING COMMUNITY LEADERS

The survey of community leaders began with a presentation held at the request of project research staff, who asked the director of the county health department to gather all individuals whom he felt would have a stake in breast cancer screening to hear about the proposed new program and research project. About 25 individuals attended the meeting in Lee County, including representatives of hospitals, radiology practices, and voluntary health organizations, along with medical practitioners and staff from the county health department.

When the group reaction to the proposal was found to be generally favorable, research staff reviewed the list of attendees and visited individuals from each of the organizations represented at the introductory meeting. Researchers visited five or six leaders individually on each of several trips to Fort Myers. A standard interview format was used to ask about existing breast screening education and community organization efforts, capacities for adopting components of the proposed program, potential barriers, and for lists of names of other leaders who should be visited. Of 80 names listed, 45 of those most frequently endorsed, representing a broad set of community groups and networks, were interviewed over a 6-month period.

Based on these interviews, it was found that (a) both professional and lay informants thought that the program components would be a benefit to them and the populations they served, (b) the mammography facilities could absorb the increased levels of screening that might result, and (c) there was an excellent volunteer base to help program staff carry out educational functions. One concern regarding the proposed program also was voiced consistently: that it might stimulate a much higher rate of screening among low-income women who would not be able to pay for screening or follow-up breast cancer treatment services and that current services could not absorb the potential surge of free care that might be requested.

POPULATION AND PROFESSIONAL SURVEYS

With the start of project funding through the National Cancer Institute in 1990, baseline household and telephone surveys were conducted, with 694 women 40 and older randomly selected to represent the entire county and with 333 other women 40 and older to represent low-income, largely African American areas of the county (Worden, Mickey, et al., 1994). Data from these surveys indicated that (a) less than half of the women throughout the county were receiving mammography screening at recommended intervals, with very low rates of screening in the lower income, African American areas (Mickey, Durski, Worden, & Danigelis, 1995; Danigelis, Roberson, et al., 1995; Danigelis, Worden, & Mickey, 1996); and (b) 95% of the women in the entire county and 75% in the low-income areas had some form of health insurance. A survey of primary care physicians indicated that they generally overestimated what proportion of their female patients got mammography screening at recommended intervals, and they considered clinical breast exam to be less effective than either mammography or breast self-exam. A survey of mammography facilities confirmed that they had the capacity to perform an increased number of mammograms that might potentially result from the proposed program.

Establishing the Lee County Breast Screening Program

DESIGN OF THE EDUCATIONAL PROGRAM

The program began early in 1991 with the recruitment of an executive director and five other staff members assigned to guide each major program component with consultation from project investigators. The executive director, Dr. McVety, had advanced degrees and experience in nursing and health care administration; most program staff had previous experience as volunteer leaders in education or service organizations. Educational program components were developed based on previous research (Worden, Mickey, et al., 1994) and were designed to address the needs of women and medical professionals providing breast cancer screening. These program components were (a) public education for women 40 and older through small-group breast-screening education presentations led by volunteers and conducted at worksites, organizations, and women's homes (Worden, Solomon, et al., 1998); in addition, mass media public service spots promoting screening were provided, and program staff assisted local media in developing news and feature stories supporting screening. (b) An office-based training protocol in clinical breast screening techniques was developed for primary care physicians, using a training team that consisted of a trainer and a simulated patient to give feedback to the physician (Warner, Solomon, Foster, Worden, & Atkins, 1993); in addition, a program was developed to improve primary care medical office systems for maintaining better patient records and sending reminders for breast screening. (c) A mammography registry protocol was developed in which reports of all mammograms and breast biopsies in the county would be entered in a computer with results of mammographic interpretations fed back to radiologists quarterly; this had never been done before on a geographic basis and would give each radiologist greater insight into his or her own performance in interpreting mammograms for breast cancer (Clark, Geller, Peluso, McVety, & Worden, 1995). Feedback from the registry would also suggest priorities for further radiologist training. Training opportunities for mammography technologists (e.g., in patient positioning and film assessment) would also be offered in the program.

USING COMMUNITY ANALYSIS DATA TO RECRUIT VOLUNTEERS

Program staff recruited several hundred volunteers to serve on the board of directors and task forces that later evolved into permanent committees and to implement program initiatives, especially in public education. The board of directors ranged from 15 to 20 members (with turnover) during the 6-year period, and five task forces and committees had between 13 and 20 members each. A total of 116 volunteers led small-group education programs, supported by a group of about five volunteers assisting in the office and others who arranged small-group education presentations. A series of annual fund-raising events involved between 10 and 60 volunteers working on each event.

Many of the initial volunteers were community leaders who had participated in the surveys conducted earlier by research staff. Monthly meetings were arranged at the outset of the program with each of these groups: (a) a board of directors to establish the Lee County Breast Screening Program as a nonprofit 501-C-3 organization; (b) a public education task force to assist project staff in promoting and implementing volunteer-led breast screening small-group education in women's organizations and worksites throughout the county; (c) a medical practitioner task force, consisting mainly of physicians, to promote office-based training in clinical breast exam and training in the use of office records and reminder systems to Lee County primary care physicians; and (d) a mammography provider task force, comprising representatives of each mammography facility, to help establish a community mammography registry and establish radiologist and radiology technologist training priorities. In several cases, members of these task forces were first asked to participate in program components as early adopters and then were asked to recommend the components to colleagues and friends as the program was diffused throughout the professional and lay communities.

USING COMMUNITY ANALYSIS DATA TO SHAPE PROGRAM PRIORITIES

Results from the 1990 baseline surveys were presented as soon as they became available to the Board of Directors and Task Forces and representatives of public health agencies in Lee County. One area of intense interest was the proportion of women who did not have sufficient health insurance coverage. Although it was generally thought among medical professionals in the community that many Lee County women did not have coverage, the baseline survey results indicated that only about 1 woman out of 10 actually lacked health insurance. When this result was confirmed by other health agency and hospital data reviews, it became apparent that the problem was actually quite manageable, and through a brainstorming session between program staff and volunteer leaders, a solution was created.

The result of this process was the formation of an advocacy task force comprising representatives of each hospital in the county, the county public health director and the director of a nonprofit public health agency, radiologists, surgeons, anesthesiologists, radiation therapists, oncologists, pathologists, and concerned board members. This is an example of a medical care and public health partnership discussed in Chapter 4. All members agreed to establish Partners in Health, a system to provide breast biopsies and treatment to women without health insurance whose incomes were at 150% of poverty level or less. It was agreed that (a) the Lee County Breast Screening Program, Inc. would raise funds to pay for diagnostic mammograms, ultrasounds, and 50% of biopsy and laboratory charges (this was about $1,100; the remainder would be donated by providers), and the program would supply a case manager to coordinate eligibility, diagnosis, and treatment; (b) surgeons, anesthesiologists, and hospitals would provide treatment for qualifying women with positive biopsies on a rotating basis as arranged by the case manager, and adjutant therapy would be supplied by radiation therapists and oncologists with donated medications from pharmaceutical companies; (c) the American Cancer Society would raise $25,000 to provide mammogram screenings to qualified women; and (d) this entire system would be tried for a year to see if it was indeed manageable.

COMMUNITY PARTICIPATION THROUGH FUND-RAISING

To support Partners in Health, it was necessary for the Lee County Breast Screening Program, Inc., to raise funds. Because this kind of activity could not be covered under the federal research grant, a development task force was formed, comprising local business leaders, directors of voluntary agencies, development directors at area hospitals, politicians, and physicians. This committee lent advice to a few volunteers who launched efforts to raise funds through local grants, donations, and events. Chief among these were annual tennis benefits and grants from local foundations and municipalities in Lee County. It took about a year to develop fund-raising skills in the group and to convince other nonprofit organizations in the county that this program served a unique purpose that was worthy of competing for contributions. However, the effort gained momentum early with the appearance of a needy client, a young mother needing a breast biopsy. Her story, told in several gatherings and through the local media, created a focus on the problem and generated an emotional appeal that caught the attention of the community.

IDENTIFYING PUBLIC EDUCATION PRIORITIES

In another use of community analysis data, public education outreach approaches were developed for African American women in low-income areas of Lee County who had been identified in the baseline survey as having extremely low levels of screening. In October 1991, program staff and researchers developed these new approaches based on a series of focus groups (Danigelis, Roberson, et al., 1995). These groups were arranged with help from the Minority Health Care Committee, a group of African American health professionals in Fort Myers established the year before to explore ways of improving health care for minority populations in Lee County. A team of eight African American volunteers was trained in leading breast screening small-group education programs, and they recruited women door to door to attend group programs offered in community rooms in largely African American housing developments in Fort Myers. At each program, women signed up for a clinical breast exam and mammogram offered at a nearby clinic. With this process of small-group education followed by clinic visits, 90% of the women eligible for screening obtained the clinical breast exams and mammograms. This was a very important effort for the program to make in the first year of its operation because it focused attention on reaching lower income women and women of color in Lee County, who are less likely to be early adopters of new interventions. Had the survey data not been available, program staff might not have identified the needs of these women as a priority and would have spent too many resources on those women who were early adopters and likely to receive regular screening anyway.

Long-Term Durability of the Program

From 1990 through 1998, the Lee County Breast Screening Program, with its staff of six and several hundred volunteers, has disseminated breast screening education to over 13,000 women and 170 physicians throughout the county, with a special emphasis on providing educational outreach to 2,400 lower income and African American women, along with financial support for screening diagnosis and treatment services. The Partners in Health collaboration has continued, with 660 women receiving diagnostic and/or treatment services through January 1998. However, the program underwent a major transition in December 1996 when funding from the National Cancer Institute came to an end, and the community was faced with supporting program components largely by itself.

STRATEGIC PLANNING FOR LONG-TERM DURABILITY

The date of the termination of federal program funding was known to program staff and volunteers several years in advance. During this time, a volunteer Strategic Planning Committee was convened to prioritize the importance of various program components to the long-term breast screening education and service needs of the community and to plan for providing support for these components. See Chapter 7 (durability planning) for further discussion of the need for early planning.

PRESERVING THE COMMUNITY MAMMOGRAPHY REGISTRY

One component that gained importance for the medical community over the course of the program was the Community Mammography Registry. When established in 1991 as the first geographically based mammography and pathology registry, the 38 radiologists in Lee County supported it on an experimental basis (Clark et al., 1995). However, under the recent Mammography Quality Standards Act, the federal government has placed a higher priority on monitoring quality assurance information. To establish funding for the Community Mammography Registry, a finance subcommittee was formed within the Mammography Providers Committee that assessed each participating radiology practice or hospital system for a portion of the expenses to operate the registry. As part of a follow-up research grant conducted by the project investigators, 10% of staff salaries and facility costs are provided by the research project so researchers can access registry data for evaluation purposes.

PRESERVING PARTNERS IN HEALTH

A second component of continuing importance to the community was the Partners in Health program. The Lee County Breast Screening Program continued its annual schedule of grant application submissions and fund-raising events to earn between $50,000 and $80,000 per year to provide no-cost diagnostic services to lower income women and to continue collaboration with physicians and hospitals providing pro bono treatment to these women. The Partners in Health component was found to be important for several reasons: (a) there was no other agency that would provide support for breast cancer diagnostic or treatment services for uninsured low-income women in Lee County, and the community recognized the Lee County Breast Screening Program as a unique resource for this purpose; and (b) it was observed that having a "cause" that evoked an emotional response strengthened the community's attachment to the program. Although the breast screening education components were well supported by both professional and lay groups in the community, the willingness of the program to address the plight of uninsured women unable to cope with breast cancer resulted in much higher enthusiasm and loyalty to the overall mission of the program than could have been achieved by the education program alone. Clearly, local empowerment was enhanced (see Chapter 4).

PRESERVING PROGRAM IDENTITY

To maintain community confidence in the durability of the program beyond the period of federal funding, it was considered essential to keep up a basic minimal activity pattern of educational and fund-raising efforts supporting breast screening and Partners in Health. Public and professional educational activities were no longer promoted regularly in the community but were offered by former program staff serving as volunteers in response to requests. To maintain the program and to facilitate communications among public and professional contacts, board members, and volunteers, the part-time position of program coordinator was formed, along with a part-time Partners in Health case manager position. A part-time financial coordinator was also needed to maintain fiscal records for the organization. A portion of the program coordinator position was paid through the follow-up research grant to ensure that research data on program progress were made available for evaluation purposes. Because the program accomplished most of its professional and public education goals when fully funded from federal sources, requests for these services diminished, except in October and April, which are cancer awareness months. During those months, the program coordinator, board members, and other volunteers usually put forth extra effort to provide information about breast cancer and the program to local media and community groups, and a semiannual newsletter has been sent in April and October to keep the community aware of program activity.

Perhaps the most innovative strategic plan involved making a long-term financial investment to ease the transition to community support and ownership for the program after federal funding expired. With 4 years remaining in the federally funded project, the board of directors elected to purchase a small office building and renovate it with volunteer labor into an attractive program office. Funds from the research grant that had been going into rental fees at an office complex were used to rent the building from the board of directors. This rental income enabled the board to make regular mortgage payments. When federal program funding ended, the building was sold at a reduced price to a buyer who agreed to provide space and telephone service to the program in a portion of the building. Proceeds from this transaction provided sufficient income to pay the salaries of the program director (100%) and the public education coordinator (60%) during a 6-month period when the program made the transition from a large staff effort with full funding to a self-supported volunteer organization facilitated by a program coordinator. This period of transition went smoothly as responsibilities were redefined, with key functions of the program being maintained and the home base and telephone number of the program preserved.

The major continuing entity for ensuring durability of the Lee County Breast Screening Program has been the board of directors, with its oversight of the Partners in Health commitment by the medical community, its fund-raising priorities, and its support of the Community Mammography Registry. This board has been guided by strong leadership of former staff and board members, especially the executive director and the public education coordinator, and a radiologist who is well known in the community and has served as a board member since 1991 and as president for several years; these individuals have a deep commitment to ensuring that the key components of the program will be continued. This effort includes constant nurturing of the fund-raising base by submitting grant applications each year to long-term supporters and by sponsoring annual fund-raising events in which people with the ability to pay help those who cannot pay to get diagnoses and treatment for breast cancer.

A Final Point

The formal evaluation of this community program will entail the analysis and interpretation of follow-up surveys conducted in 1997 to determine whether it increased breast screening among women in Lee County compared to women in the comparison community, with results expected by mid-1998. However, in one sense the program already has had a positive impact on the Lee County community. During the course of 6 years, the program has encouraged the participation of hundreds of lay volunteers and hundreds of physicians, a group of hospitals that grew from four to six during the period, county and city governments, and a score of public and voluntary health agencies, private foundations, and local businesses. Through Partners in Health, the program has brought strangers and competitors together to work on a common problem, providing essential health care to low-income women. In this extension of the original project design, community participation (as suggested by Schwab & Syme, 1997) has already benefited at least 660 women receiving help from Partners in Health and has also equipped the community with the motivation and skills to address problems through cooperative action.

CHAPTER 4

A Five-Stage Community Organization Model for Health Promotion

Empowerment and Partnership Strategies

NEIL BRACHT

LEE KINGSBURY

CHRIS RISSEL

In Chapter 2, the theoretical foundations for understanding social change at the community level are presented. This is followed in Chapter 3 with the tools and strategies for conducting a comprehensive community needs assessment. The focus of this chapter is on the applied process of mobilizing citizens and organizations to facilitate the empowerment of communities for effective health and social improvement. Collaboration is fostered and local empowerment is realized through the marshalling of community interest, talent, and resources. Organizers (both professional and lay) bring together networks of government and voluntary groups to plan and implement health program goals and objectives.

The authors present a five-stage model of organizing for health promotion that builds on principles developed through years of field experience and research in many disciplines. In addition to the reported experiences of numerous community demonstrations, some of the more important influences that have shaped the model's development include (a) the authors' own applied community organization work, (b) general principles of social and community change, (c) elements of organizational development and strategic planning, and (d) community empowerment theory.

As our understanding of the nature of health and its determinants broadens, so also does our appreciation of the importance of a broader community perspective, one in which many public and private entities have a stake or that can affect the community's health. New partnerships are forming between community members, health care providers, public health officials, and nontraditional participants (e.g., business, labor, religious groups). These partnerships have the potential to achieve public health goals. However, they leave questions about the role of citizen involvement and empowerment. A more detailed discussion of these emerging issues and partnerships is found in Part II, Chapter 12.

Regardless of the nature or form that health promotion collaborations take in the future, the lessons of the past converge to provide one clear message: individuals and groups in communities need to feel in control and need to be empowered to collectively control factors that influence health and well-being. Because of the central importance of this theory base, the authors first recap the guiding principles of empowerment and ownership. Then, as in the first edition, the five-stage model (updated) is presented as a guide for health action. The chapter is followed by a case study of a rural community organization project (Northland). Here, the lessons of best community practice are integrated with the five-stage model in the context of a community-based alcohol intervention program.

Community Organization

Background and Definition

The evolution of community organization practice and methods covers a period of some 75 years. Its history is documented by several writers, particularly from the social work field, where community organization has been taught and researched as an area of professional practice since the 1940s (Cox, Erlich, Rothman, & Tropman, 1979; Kramer & Specht, 1975). Principles of community organization draw from national and international experience in a wide range of disciplines. Prominent among these are urban and rural sociology, social work, community psychology, health education, anthropology, international community development, consumer and union advocacy, and university agricultural extension services. Documents produced by the United Nations began referring to the field of "community development" in the 1950s. The terms *community organization* and *development* are often interchangeable. Numerous community organization efforts in the United States were undertaken in the 1960s and 1970s as a result of federal funding for antipoverty projects (for example, neighborhood community health centers). By the 1980s and 1990s, Rothman's three community organization models had become fundamental components of the mushrooming community-based health promotion movement (see Table 4.1).

The community organization approach is not new to public health. Public health issues were early targets for community organization and social reform (Miller, 1976). The work of charity organization societies and settlement houses, for example, included health and environmental protection efforts. Block committees of local mothers (e.g., Hull House in Chicago) were organized in support of early maternal and child health clinics. The National Citizens' Committee on Prevention of Tuberculosis worked closely with public health professionals to combat infectious diseases during this period. The National Mental Hygiene movement of the 1930s was a citizen-

TABLE 4.1 Three Models of Community Organization Practice According to Selected Practice Variables

	Model A (Locality Development)	Model B (Social Planning)	Model C (Social Action)
Categories of community action	self-help; community capacity and integration (process goals)	problem solving with regard to substantive community problems (task goals)	shifting of power relationships and resources; basic institutional change (task or process goals)

SOURCE: Rothman's (1979) comprehensive table of variables.

based group that also supported the work of professional associations. Rosen (1974), a noted public health historian, has written about the early interrelationship between social welfare and public health services:

> To a large extent the history of social medicine is also the history of social policy (welfare). . . . The roots of social medicine are to be found in organized social work. It was here that medicine and social science found a common ground for action in the prevention of tuberculosis, securing better housing and work conditions. (p. 112)

For many years, Rothman's (1979) three models of community organization practice provided some of the most useful conceptualizations for understanding various approaches to organizing (see Table 4.1). More recently, Rothman (1996) has elaborated on the interaction and overlap between these models and their applications for practitioners. His observations ring true to organizers and researchers involved in recent communitywide health promotion projects. Comprehensive approaches require strategies of *locality development* with broad community participation and citizen ownership. Considerable *social planning* technology is used in community needs assessment and analysis work. Professional planners are frequently involved in assisting communities and citizens to determine needs and intervention strategies. Increasingly, social policy, legislation, and advocacy initiatives (such as campaigns for nonsmokers' rights and/or state legal action against the tobacco industry, such as in Minnesota) are being used in *social action* orientations. The National Cancer Institute's smoking prevention project (ASSIST) strongly endorses a policy advocacy strategy.

Stimulation or activation of the community is a process whereby a community (a) becomes aware of a condition or problem that exists within a community, (b) identifies that condition as a priority of community action, (c) institutes steps to change the condition, and (d) establishes structures to implement and maintain program solutions. Community activation requires not only the creation or presence of an issue, but also the identification and activation of community groups and individuals to deal with the issue.

The organizing process is a critical aspect of health action and is a kind of "glue" that maintains citizen interest, nourishes participation in programs, and encourages support for long-term maintenance of successful intervention efforts. Because the term *community organization* has several meanings and definitions, we will, for purposes of consistency and clarity, use the following definition:

> Community organization is a planned process to activate a community to use its own social structures and any available resources to accomplish community goals that are decided on primarily by community representatives and that are generally consistent with local values. Purposive social change interventions are organized primarily by individuals, groups, or organizations from within the community to attain and then sustain community improvements and/or new opportunities.

Important aspects of the process of community and citizen involvement are community ownership and empowerment. Communities must shape their own program directions and emerge with the necessary skills and resources to manage continued efforts. Community representatives clearly have a choice as to whether to participate in health demonstrations that originate from professionals outside the community. Some professionals are even experimenting with assisting community groups to design their own evaluation tools and measures (Maltrud, Polacsek, & Wallerstein, 1997).

Community organizers, often referred to as local field directors, need to have the experience and skill to work with diverse groups and coalitions. They should have a basic understanding of community change processes and bring proven management experience to the local effort. Good facilitation and listening skills are also important. Selection of the local field director should, when possible, be done in consultation with the citizen leaders of the coalition or community board. This is but one way of empowering communities. See Figure 4.1 for a brief summary of knowledge and skills desired in a project field director. Of course, this is not an exhaustive list.

EMPOWERMENT: THEORY AND PRACTICE

Empowerment is a central construct for health promotion. For example, the World Health Organization (1986) defined *health promotion* in a document known as the Ottawa Charter as "the process of enabling people to increase control over, and to improve, their health" (p. 1). This definition suggests a picture of health promotion as a dynamic process or series of events and strategies that must necessarily involve consumers and consumer ownership of the process.

Empowerment has been defined in many ways. We prefer to make a distinction between psychological and community empowerment, in line with major differences between the subjective perception of greater control and the objective reality of greater power following a reallocation of resources (Rissel, 1994). The distinction is an important one. Psychological empowerment can be defined as a subjective feeling of greater control over one's own life that an individual experiences following active membership in groups or organizations. Psychological empowerment may occur without participation in collective political action and is assessed with the individual as the unit of analysis. The distinction between active membership in groups and participation in collective action lies in the nature and amount of activism of the group. If a group or organization does not act collectively to increase its members' resources (for example, a soccer club) then active membership does not constitute collective political or social action. The distinction is subtle and

Knowledge
- Community change process
- Local history, values, resources

Skill and Experience
- Network or communitywide approach
- Management or evaluative orientation

Interpersonal
- Facilitator or energizer
- Conflict resolution

Figure 4.1. Competencies of Local Organizer

the status of the group may change if the group or organization begins to seek to expand its influence.

Community empowerment is a state that communities or community subgroups may attain. It can be considered as defined by participation in collective political action that results in (a) a raised level of psychological empowerment and (b) the achievement of some redistribution of resources or decision making sought by a community or subgroup.

Community participation has been directly linked to empowerment as the principal mechanism by which individuals and groups become empowered and as a means of promoting healthier individuals, communities, and environments (Wallerstein, 1993; World Health Organization, 1991). Participation facilitates psychological empowerment by developing personal efficacy, developing a sense of group action, developing a critical understanding of social power relationships, and developing a willingness to participate in collective action. Psychological empowerment and community empowerment are linked through the logical expectation that there ought to be empowered individuals within an empowered community. It is possible that an empowered community facilitates the psychological empowerment of individuals. On the other hand, the collective actions of psychologically empowered individuals can lead to an empowered community. Alternatively, psychological empowerment and community empowerment may be two independent constructs that do not overlap.

Community empowerment is linked with community by definition. For there to be an empowered community, "community" must exist. Psychological empowerment is linked to community because "sense of community" has been found to enhance citizen participation in groups and organizations and in social action, as well as sense of personal power to influence people and events (Chavis & Wandersman, 1990). By enhancing participation in collective action, a raised sense of community within a community contributes to the likelihood that the community is empowered. It might be expected that groups with actual control over resources have a high level of reported psychological empowerment, although the reverse is not necessarily true. For example, a neighborhood association that is successful in zoning land into a children's park or reducing traffic speed through local streets is likely to feel psychologically empowered. Another neighborhood group that has a high level of active membership and feelings of psychological empowerment among members may not have been successful in acquiring resources for their community or successfully influencing a public decision-making process. Groups with high levels of reported psychological empowerment may not have much control over resources.

THE PROCESS OF EMPOWERMENT AND PARTICIPATION

Several authors have identified the work of Alinsky (1946), Friere (1973), and Rothman (1979) as the intellectual and practical basis of the concept of community empowerment (Eng, Salmon, & Mullan, 1992; Fahlberg, Poulin, Girdano, & Dusek, 1991; Gibson, 1991; Swift & Levin, 1987; Wallerstein, 1992; Wallerstein & Bernstein, 1988). Commonalities across these descriptions of empowerment include processes of personal development, participation, consciousness-raising (for example, increasing awareness of social power relationships), and social action.

Because community development or organization is the means by which communities or groups might become empowered, the community health development continuum, developed almost simultaneously on two continents (Jackson, Mitchell, & Wright, 1989; Labonte, 1989a, 1989b), is a useful schema for representing the psychological and community empowerment process. The potential for community empowerment is maximized as the focus shifts from the individual to collective social action (see Figure 4.2), although the process need not be simply linear, with one stage automatically following the other. For example, personal development might follow participation in an organization, or support groups might emerge following issue identification activities.

The process of community empowerment begins with an assumption that a power deficit or an unattended social problem exists, despite the presence of some competencies. By contrast, an empowered community logically should include groups of individuals who have a raised sense of empowerment. Psychological empowerment may require some individual personal development, such as increases in self-esteem or self-efficacy (Bandura, 1986), at least to the point where that individual is willing and able to join a group and function effectively within it.

Joining mutual support, self-help, or action groups (whether formal or informal) builds and expands social networks and provides an opportunity for a personal mentor (Kieffer, 1984) or group to support a personal development process. At the same time, individuals may become more critically aware of how political structures operate and affect them and their subgroups, or this critical consciousness or awareness may develop through participation in a group or other mediating social structure. Participation in and influence of a group or organization is an important stage of both psychological and community empowerment (Florin & Wandersman, 1990; Green, 1986). It is often the means by which people learn skills that may then be able to transfer to other situations (Wandersman, 1981) and how communities develop their problem-solving capacity (Batten, 1967).

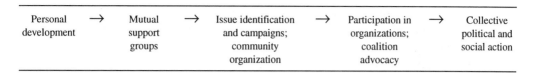

| Personal development | → | Mutual support groups | → | Issue identification and campaigns; community organization | → | Participation in organizations; coalition advocacy | → | Collective political and social action |

Figure 4.2. Community Development Stages for Maximizing Community Empowerment Potential
SOURCE: Adapted from Jackson et al., 1989; Labonte, 1989a, 1989b.

Participation in collective action is also fundamental to the successful redistribution of resources, which is necessary before a community or community subgroup can be said to be empowered. The emphasis on community action as a core component of community empowerment (Brown, 1991) is also consistent with the principles of health promotion (Miner & Ward, 1992) and voluntary organizations (O'Connell, 1978). Issues being addressed by the group or community should be or have been identified by the group. Ideally, the outcome of the community empowerment process is a greater degree of psychological empowerment among community members than before the process, as well as an actual increase in control over resources.

A visual representation of the preceding discussion of the components of community empowerment is presented in Figure 4.3. It can be seen that psychological empowerment plus collective political or social action plus an actual increase in control over resources (to some degree) constitute an empowered community. A feedback mechanism is shown. The degree of success in gaining control over resources should influence the level of psychological empowerment of participants. Also, the process of empowerment might positively or negatively affect health, depending on the focus of the community organizing and empowerment activities. The specificity of the focus of collective action and its consequences for health is an argument that community empowerment is topic-specific and not a general all-inclusive construct. In Australia, a national gun control lobby was established following a mass shooting at a shopping center in Strathfield, Sydney in 1991. Despite considerable activity, it was only after another gun massacre (in Port Arthur, Tasmania) that the background research on state gun laws and the advocacy of this group influenced strong national gun control legislation in 1996 (Peters, 1996).

Putting the continuum of community development into practice can be facilitated through the application of the five stages of community organization. Once individuals are able to work in groups to address issues they identify, then the first stage of community organizing—community analysis—can begin. Psychological empowerment may result through the implementation of programs and, depending on the nature and outcomes of these programs, may lead to community empowerment.

The Five Stages of Organizing: A Community Health Promotion Process

What follows is a description of a five-stage community organizing process (see Figure 4.4). Each stage has several key elements. Citizen involvement is possible and recommended at all stages. As

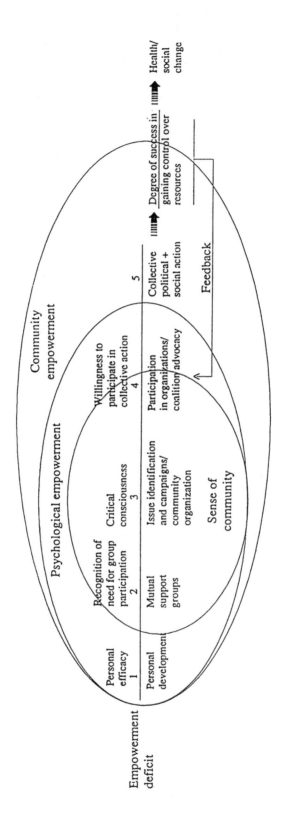

Figure 4.3. Model of the Critical Components of Psychological and Community Empowerment

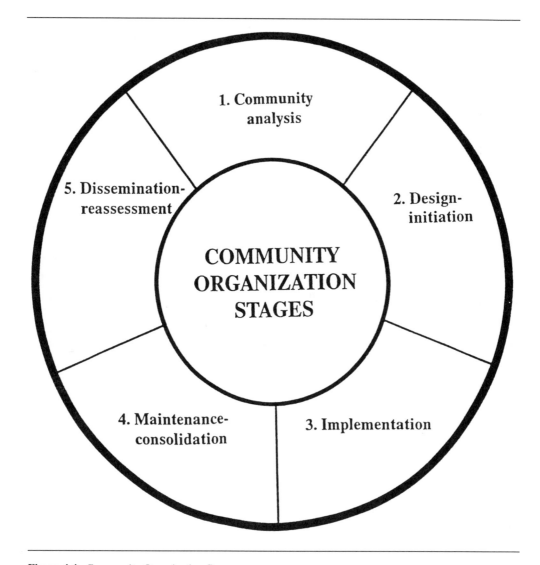

Figure 4.4. Community Organization Stages

mentioned earlier, organizing work is a dynamic process. The overlapping of these stages is common, and some of the tasks or key elements may need to be repeated. For example, planning for maintenance and/or durability must begin early in the analysis and design phase and then must be reassessed during both the maintenance and dissemination stages.

STAGE 1: COMMUNITY ANALYSIS OR ASSESSMENT

Successful implementation of communitywide health promotion and intervention programs depends in large part on two interrelated sets of activities: first, accurate analysis and understanding of a community's needs, resources, social structure, and values, and second, early citizen leader and organizational involvement to build collaborative partnerships and facilitate broad community participation. This latter activity ensures that programs are designed to reflect community values and encourage long-term community ownership. *Assessing community capacity to support a project, identifying potential barriers that exist,* and *evaluating community readiness for involvement* are key areas of the community analysis. A detailed methodology for community analysis or assessment is described in Chapter 3. We highlight only the major steps here.

Key Elements

1. Define the community. One of the first tasks should be to determine the geographic focus or target group of the project. As discussed in Chapters 2 and 3, the term *community* has different meanings and interpretations. Will the project focus on a neighborhood, a city, a region, or nation? Clarity about community boundaries or "sense of community" is critical. Typically, organizers will want to decide on the community target area after consulting with representatives from major social institutions or sectors such as education, health, recreation, business, religious, media, and civic organizations and government. It is helpful to solicit information on past community organization efforts, their successes, failures, and decision-making processes. If more than one community is involved, the patterns of social interaction and cooperative decision making should be discerned. Past studies completed in the community may assist in this process.

2. Collect data. Community analysis involves the collection and analysis of a variety of data (see Chapter 3). The compilation of a comprehensive community profile of health and demographic information is quite helpful. This community profile should include information on community resources, history, and readiness for action. A sample community analysis profile is presented in the Lee County case study that follows Chapter 3.

Organizers must determine what citizens perceive as community needs and must identify who can get things done, who is ready to provide resources, who needs to be involved in decision making, and who may be opposed to health promotion efforts. Gathering the variety of data necessary requires numerous personal contacts, but in the process the groundwork for citizen mobilization begins. The purpose of key informant interviews is shown in Table 4.2.

3. Assess community capacity. What are the community forces that will support change? As mentioned earlier, the current level of health promotion activity in the community and the potential for increasing activity need to be assessed and summarized. This summary should provide concise information on current programs, identify key leaders or influential people or groups within each of the various community sectors (e.g., school, business) and describe organizational structure(s), available skilled personnel, programmatic and financial resources, and the general feasibility of focusing the community's interest on a particular health agenda. Based on this assessment of potential, the types of resources needed to develop an adequate community program are defined for each community sector, as are the types of actions needed to increase capacity. Identification of potential collaborating organizations, programs, and individuals is emphasized.

TABLE 4.2 The Purpose of Key Informant Interviews

- To identify data sources that can be used in site analysis
- To verify and help make sense of information gathered from other sources
- To provide important information that is not easily captured in statistics or documents
- To identify and provide access to other key community informants who should be interviewed

---

4. Assess community barriers. An analysis of potential barriers or restraining forces is crucial to good planning. Organizers should look for unique local characteristics and customs that could inhibit interventions. Ethnic dietary patterns, for example, may need to be understood if nutrition interventions are to be designed successfully. Will voluntary organizations with their own agendas cooperate with a new program effort? Do people believe they can make changes? What is the extent of grassroots citizen involvement in decision making? Historically, has this community been supportive or resistant to changes?

The initiation of a change process can be viewed as creating its own barriers. As Nix (1978) states, resistance to change is a normal human reaction. He defines five kinds of changes people frequently resist:

- changes not clearly understood,
- changes they or their representatives had no part in bringing about,
- changes that threaten their vested interest and security,
- changes advocated by those they do not like or trust, and
- changes that do not fit into the cultural values of the community.

After conditions are identified that might inhibit interventions, community organizers need to be proactive in suggesting alternative methods and strategies to cope with or respond to known areas of resistance.

5. Assess readiness for change. How ready a community may be for change will influence program planning. Information previously collected during assessment of community capacity and barriers will help here. The organizing group will want to assess the intensity of community interest, the urgency of the problem as perceived by key influentials, and the general awareness levels of community members. How receptive are top decision makers? How has the community reacted to similar issues or past community organizing efforts?

6. Synthesize data and set priorities. Once data have been gathered from all the above sources, a summary report should be compiled. Typically this summary includes overall social and health data, community needs, current levels of activity, barriers, potential resources, and readiness for health promotion. Researchers and citizens must analyze the data carefully to make appropriate plans and choices. Ideally, community members should review the profile, thoroughly discuss all of the information and ideas, and set priorities. A consensus decision-making meeting involving key community leaders is most often used for synthesizing ideas and setting priorities.

STAGE 2: DESIGN AND INITIATION

Following community analysis and the identification of local priorities, the design aspects for a community intervention begin to emerge. Concurrently, formal activities to mobilize citizens begin with the establishment of a structure to elicit and/or coordinate broad citizen support and involvement (informal mobilization of selected citizens began during the analysis stage). As decisions are being made about design and organizational structure, other actions are under way, including identifying individuals who may wish to participate in a community board, coalition, or similar structure; contacting individuals to serve on the board or solicit interest; developing working relationships between the project and various collaborating public and private groups; and legitimating the board's activities within the community. Focus groups (Krueger, 1988) can be useful in helping to decide some aspects of design and intervention stages.

Key Elements

1. Establish a core planning group and select a local organizer or coordinator. Green and McAlister (1984) have described the extensive planning and coordination efforts that community-wide health promotion programs require. A core group or executive committee is usually responsible for long-term planning. This group consists of five to eight interested members who make a commitment to plan and participate in the administration of the project. The group's responsibilities may include calling public attention to the data analysis and identified needs, writing a mission statement, choosing the organization's likely structure, selecting a coordinator, and identifying and recruiting board members.

The experience and skill of the lead coordinator or organizer is extremely important to program success. The person employed for this purpose must understand how change occurs in communities and must be knowledgeable about local history and values. A local resident or professional is generally preferred. Past experience in facilitating organizational collaboration, including good management skills, is critical. At the interpersonal level, one looks for an energetic, experienced person with good listening and conflict-resolution skills. Usually paid health professionals are employed to facilitate the work of a citizen group (see summary in Figure 4.1).

2. Choose an organizational structure. There are several alternative structures for organizing community involvement and participation, including advisory board, council, coalition, lead agency, informal network, and grassroots or advocacy movements. These structures are described in more detail in Chapter 7 (which deals with durability). Three structures (coalition, board, and grassroots) are briefly discussed below. The type of structure chosen depends on the community culture, history, and past decision-making style, but successful programs are likely to use parts from several organizing models. Choice of organizational structure usually rests with the community and its representatives. However, some funding agencies often proscribe in advance the community structure most preferred or recommended (e.g., coalition). This is risky; one model cannot fit all communities.

An important lesson to be learned from earlier demonstration projects is that citizen-based structures are dynamic. Often they evolve into new or modified arrangements. Organizing structures can be combined to suit local conditions. New structures can emerge. Because of the importance of structure, we provide a more substantive discussion of this key element before continuing on with other elements of the design and initiation stage. Three major organizing structures are discussed:

1. Citizen coalitions
2. Community boards and task forces
3. Grassroots organization or network

1. COALITIONS

The coalition (an alliance of several community groups and/or health organizations) has become an increasingly popular vehicle for implementing community health promotion efforts. *Coalition* has been defined as "an organization of individuals representing diverse organizations, factions or constituencies who agree to work together in order to achieve a common goal" (Feighery, Rogers, Thompson, & Bracht, 1992, p. 1). In their excellent review of the literature on coalitions, Butterfoss, Goodman, and Wandersman (1993) provide a detailed look at coalition formation, implementation, maintenance, and outcomes. Coalitions serve multiple functions in a health promotion program, including acting as direct links from outside agencies to communities, enhancing ownership and continuation of programs, and assisting in mobilizing community residents and resources to achieve program objectives. Coalitions can also influence the public policy process, and coalition action may raise or lower the importance of public issues (Herman, Wolfson, & Forster, 1993).

One study of coalition effectiveness is a 5-year study of drug use prevention funded by the Center for Substance Abuse Prevention (ISA Associates, 1992). Involving over 200 coalitions across the United States, this study examined the relationship of coalition effectiveness and such factors as coalition type, age of coalition, and population density. Secondary factors of interest include the assessment of the socioeconomic climate, size and composition of membership, membership recruitment, organizational structure, and coalition dynamics.

The coalition model uses existing organizations to address community issues. The process of building a coalition involves constructing linkages among existing organizations, groups, and agencies. Coalitions often arise in response to a specific issue or unmet need. The major advantage of a coalition is that it involves a breadth and diversity of membership that may make for strange bedfellows but cuts across ideologies and constituencies. The leaders of each organization are likely to become more committed as the scope of the coalition's membership increases. If existing coalitions can be tapped, much of the work and time of recruitment of community leaders and networking between community factions can be minimized. The coalition can minimize jealousy between organizations if all members of the coalition receive equal credit for achievements.

Carlyn and Bracht (1995) reviewed the literature on coalition effectiveness and found the functions listed in Table 4.3 important to overall coalition productivity.

Leadership was mentioned most frequently as the most important function of coalition effectiveness. Coalitions by their nature are complex and fragile entities. Skilled leaders are required to make them effective organizing structures.

TABLE 4.3 Factors and Skills Important to the Effectiveness of Partnerships and Coalitions

Factor or Skill	Definition
Leadership	The extent to which coalitions have one or more members who are well respected and experienced in organizing group activities, garnering resources, facilitating discussion, motivating others, negotiating, and recruiting new members
Management	The extent to which coalitions have the expertise to effectively manage the meeting logistics, resources, and operations of the coalition.
Communication	The degree to which written and verbal communications among coalition members, committee and task force members, staff, and individuals outside the coalition have been clear, timely, and effective.
Conflict resolution	The degree to which friction and tensions arising from turf issues, different personalities, or competing interests of coalition members have been effectively resolved.
Perception of fairness	The extent to which coalition members perceive that they are being treated equitably and the different organizations in the coalition are contributing their fair share in terms of resources and/or work.
Shared decision making	The degree of influence that coalition members have in determining the policies and actions of the statewide coalitions and the amount of authority coalition representatives have to make decisions on behalf of the organizations they represent.
Perceived benefits versus costs	The degree to which individual members and member organizations on state and local coalitions believe the time they have served has been worthwhile.

2. COMMUNITY BOARDS AND TASK FORCES

The board leadership model brings together community leaders identified as necessary for achieving project goals. Generally, leaders from diverse segments of the community are brought together to work toward the common goal. This approach is appropriate in settings in which the community relies on key individuals from different community segments to manage public affairs and initiate program change. When an issue arises, a few key individuals tap into and energize existing informal networks to mobilize community action. This approach can be used in communities where the leaders have previously worked well together and represent a wide range of community organizations, groups, and interests.

The support of high-profile persons, which leaders are likely to be, may contribute to a bandwagon effect throughout the community. Involvement of leaders is likely to contribute to the program's legitimacy and may rally local resources.

3. GRASSROOTS ORGANIZING AND STRUCTURES

According to Wittig (1996), grassroots organizing "is viewed as a local form of collective action by community members employing various techniques, primarily as strategies for addressing the root causes of social problems" (p. 4). Although grassroots activism can be seen as a part of social movements, social movements generally develop higher levels of coordination in which many local groups may work together on a single issue. Grassroots organizing is similar to the notion of locality development described by Rothman (1979), with the group leaders, issues, and subsequent strategies identified by members.

Most of the prominent advocates of community grassroots organizing see it as the beginnings of social change. The committed collective action of a small group of people can begin processes that improve the conditions of communities (Bettencourt, 1996). For example, in an area of Sydney with a large concentration of Southeast Asian refugees, a small group of Khmer community health workers living and working in the area agreed that the basic hygiene standards of many of the refugees from the remote villages of Cambodia needed to be improved. They organized sufficient funding for the production of culturally appropriate resources and a Khmer language video that proved to be enormously popular. Resources and the video were distributed using community networks. An evaluation reported that two thirds of the local population had seen the video and that there was an observable improvement in hygiene standards (Rissel, 1992).

One study of the factors associated with participation in rural grassroots task forces for the prevention of alcohol use among young adolescents found that members were likely to participate more in the task forces if they were relative newcomers to the community and if they got satisfaction from their participation (Rissel, Finnegan, Wolfson, & Perry, 1995). These results also suggested that satisfaction with being a task force member can be increased through the democratic operation of the task forces and processes that maximize the amount of control and ownership each member feels, thus increasing the likelihood that the member agrees with the direction of the task force. Other studies have found that a strong and supportive leader, as well as one familiar to members, is a significant factor in increasing participation in and viability of community organizations (Feighery et al., 1992).

One of the noteworthy features of grassroots organizations is that initiators and leaders are not professionals whose job it is to run a program or chair a meeting. Grassroots activity can be started by anyone with an issue to address and an ability to communicate a message. This communication is often more effective when it is a personally held belief rather than simply part of the job.

We now return to further discussion of the key elements in the design and initiation phase.

3. Identify and recruit organization members. Many key informants contacted in the community analysis phase can be recruited for the implementation phase. Generally, these representatives should be people who can speak and make decisions for the organizations or people they represent. Enlisting people from differing backgrounds and interests provides creative thinking and fresh approaches to community change. Citizen groups need members who are positive thinkers—enthusiastic people who believe in the mission of the project and who enjoy a challenge. Experienced advocates may be required for certain policy change initiatives.

4. Define the organization's mission and goals. A mission statement provides the organization or project with its goal and objectives. It should concisely and briefly communicate what is to be achieved. (An example of a mission/goal statement is presented in Table 4.4.)

5. Clarify roles and responsibilities of citizen or coalition members, staff, and volunteers. Defining roles and responsibilities for individual board and task force members, organizations,

TABLE 4.4 Forsyth County Cancer Screening Project

Project goal
  To improve breast and cervical cancer screening among underserved women aged 40 and older.

Project objective
  To reduce the burden of breast and cervical cancer among these women by improving knowledge, attitudes, and participation in cancer screening.

---

volunteers, and staff will help establish smooth working relationships. Roles can be clarified and assigned in keeping with individual abilities, interests, and expectations. Written or verbal job descriptions or agreements are often used by both volunteers and organizational staff to specify the length of the commitment, training opportunities available, specific tasks and functions, support from staff, personal expectations, and organizational commitment, if any. A responsibility charting form (modified) used by staff in the National Cancer Institute's ASSIST project is shown in Table 4.5.

Citizen boards' members, along with paid professionals, usually share the overall responsibilities in planning and implementing communitywide intervention activities. Typical tasks include electing officers; approving budgets; selecting program office site; reviewing data; writing, approving, and prioritizing goals and objectives; developing annual action plans and disseminating information about them; coordinating programs; conducting public awareness campaigns; and recruiting additional volunteers to serve on task forces and to review evaluation plans. Issues of the board's legal liability may surface. State laws and practices regarding such liability should be reviewed. Organizing task forces or work groups is one way to broaden the base of community support and ownership in the project. Task forces address specific components of the project. Members of the target population should be included on task forces. Community task forces usually require staff support. Typically, a citizen board member will chair a task force, but, with few exceptions, paid staff are necessary to attend to daily activities and to provide technical support and professional consultation.

6. Provide training and recognition. Effective citizen and volunteer involvement includes training and skill development. Professional organizers sometimes fear loss of control in turning over some intervention work to citizen task forces, but this is a critical step in community empowerment. With appropriate information and guidance, citizens can successfully form partnerships with health professionals to plan and conduct programs for their community. In the process of learning new skills themselves, citizen ownership is enhanced. Training helps members increase confidence about their abilities and contributes to community projects. Orientation and training may take many forms (e.g., weekend retreats, training sessions during board meetings). Ongoing education yields long-term benefits, including the development of new leadership to incorporate and sustain program efforts in the community. Recognition of early program planning successes and associated personal accomplishments builds pride, raises morale, boosts the awareness of the organization, and maintains better understanding, interest, and commitment. Project or professional staff need to recognize the small successes of each program component and continually create different ways to reinforce and reward people.

TABLE 4.5 Responsibility Charting

	Project and/or Field Director	Field Staff	Coalition or Board	Steering Committee	Other
1. Determine goals and priorities					
2. Design strategies and programs					
3. Decide on programs for implementation					
4. Identify resources for program					
5. Community and public relations					
6. Program administration					
7. Recruit new coalition members					
8. Chair meetings and prepare agendas					
9. Conduct training and determine scope of work					
10. Staff hiring					
11. Develop personnel policies, bylaws					
12. Recruit volunteers					
13. Maintain communication					
14. Prepare and approve budget					
15. Design evaluation strategy(ies)					
16. Purchases (materials and equipment)					
17. Update community analysis					
18. Plan for durability					
19. Review progress, perform evaluations					
20. Disseminate results					
Other Tasks:					

STAGE 3: IMPLEMENTATION

Implementation turns theory and ideas into action, translating design into effectively operating programs. Professionals and citizens are mobilized and involved in the planning of a sequential set of activities to accomplish their mission. Written action plans have been shown to be a critical forerunner of successful change efforts (Fawcett, Lewis, et al., 1997). They also maximize the use of available community resources in the plan and adapt to local constraints and values. Intervention cost estimates should be included, along with time frames. The case illustrations presented in this book provide useful information about a wide range of health promotion interventions, as well as obstacles to implementation.

Key Elements

1. Determine priority intervention activities. Review existing services and policies and identify gaps. Choose areas that need strengthening. Thoroughly analyze the pros and cons of each possible activity. What will be most and least acceptable to the community and target group? What is most likely to succeed, to fail? To change community health behavior, more than periodic or "one-shot" program interventions are required. A comprehensive and coordinated effort using multiple strategies that have the potential to influence community norms widely is necessary (Farquhar, Flora, & Good, 1985). Activities must provide people with health information and opportunities to make and practice healthful choices as well as to develop community support for these choices in the form of economic incentives and policies that promote healthy choices. Whether the choice is to develop new activities where gaps exist or to strengthen existing activities, combining multiple strategies in a community has a synergistic effect; each component complements and reinforces the others.

2. Develop a sequential work plan. Developing a practical plan of work will include both short-term problem solving and long-term planning. Some community members may want to rush the process. There is a tendency to want to "jump in with both feet." Organizers will need to channel enthusiasm, helping task forces and work groups to select, evaluate, and modify incremental implementation steps according to community needs, perceptions, and overall program protocols.

3. Generate broad citizen participation. Throughout the implementation process, there must be a continuing effort to reach out to people and encourage their participation. Special care must be taken in involving minority communities. Interviews of community minority participants shed much light on current difficulties with collaboration (Koné & Sullivan, 1998). Koné and Sullivan also reflect on the need for increasing cultural competence among majority professionals. Not all people who can be helpful need be regular members of the coalition. People can be recruited for time-limited special efforts (e.g., working on a legislative campaign only or completing specific tasks).

4. Plan media interventions. Determine incentives that will encourage program participation and develop a media plan. Consider the target group and carefully design media events and promotional activities. Sophisticated social marketing and media campaigns may require technical or professional experts. Integrate community values into the programs, materials, and messages. No matter how good an intervention looks on paper or in the literature, when it is implemented in a community it must speak that community's language (Vincent, Clearle, Johnson, & Sharpe, 1988). The approaches and messages must be acceptable to the community. Ramirez (1997) has developed a most useful training manual on mass media messages and community outreach targeted for Latino populations. Similar guides have been created for other minority population groups. Community leaders should be encouraged to incorporate local values and symbols into program components. (See Chapter 5 for more detailed information on mass media planning.)

5. Obtain resource support. This task entails identifying and involving all the appropriate people whose endorsement or collaboration is needed to ensure success. Engage staff and volunteers who are willing to spend concentrated time on the many details that need attention in carrying out the activity. Adequate finances for instructors, facilities, and equipment need to be determined. Cost associated with each intervention activity should be estimated. Develop a budget, consider funding options, and locate potential sources of support, both in kind and financial.

6. Provide a system for intervention monitoring feedback. Select criteria to measure intervention effectiveness (Fawcett, Francisco, et al., 1995; Fawcett, Paine-Andrews, et al., 1996). Develop data collection methods and protocols for both process and outcome measures (also see Chapter 6). Remember, evaluation plans need to be in proportion to the duration and size of the intervention. Determine how participants, supporting organizations, and the community at large will be informed of the project's accomplishments (newsletters, public forums, and so on). Reinforce the work and progress of committees and intervention task forces with periodic feedback on selected areas of progress. Engage community participants early in thinking about issues of durability (see Chapter 7).

STAGE 4: PROGRAM MAINTENANCE—CONSOLIDATION

During this stage, community members and staff gain experience and success with the program. Problems in implementation have been encountered but have, hopefully, been dealt with successfully. The organization is developing a solid foundation in the community, and interventions are gaining acceptance. Program elements are being more fully incorporated into the established structures of the community, and community ownership is taking place. Task forces now reassess their past efforts and determine new tasks.

Key Elements

1. Integrate intervention activities into community networks. Integrating intervention activities into established community structures creates a broad context for the adoption and maintenance of health-promoting behaviors and norms. This integration can take place early in the implementation phase or can occur later, as organizations gain confidence in program operation. Key influential people and organizations can assist in program adoption and organizational maintenance. The local community board must be active in this process.

2. Establish a positive organizational climate. A positive climate is a critical factor in promoting and maintaining successful change projects. A positive environment fosters cooperation, improves retention of staff and volunteers, and sets the stage for the development of community ownership. Good group process is developed and nurtured through an attitude of trust and openness. Staff must demonstrate trust-earning behaviors, including respect and discretion. In a positive organizational environment, people look for opportunities rather than obstacles and for strengths rather than weaknesses in one another. Mistakes are used as training opportunities, and conflicts are resolved quickly and openly.

3. Establish an ongoing recruitment plan. Turnover of volunteers and even of paid staff is to be expected in multiyear projects. To counteract this, establish a plan to identify, recruit, and involve new people in the project on an ongoing basis. Seek out new members. New sources of energy and commitment can be helpful to volunteers who may be experiencing some "burnout" characteristics.

4. Acknowledge work of volunteers. Review satisfaction levels. Consider reassignments to different tasks if requested.

STAGE 5: DISSEMINATION AND REASSESSMENT

Disseminating information on project activities and the early results from their evaluation increases visibility, communitywide acceptance, and involvement. Communities and citizens will respond to repeated, clear messages describing what has been done and what continuing effort is required to solve the problem. Messages are reinforcing when influential community individuals and organizations and decision makers are involved in their presentation. Dissemination of information, of course, occurs in all phases of community health promotion. Maintaining high visibility is essential to project maintenance.

Reassessment of activities occurs continuously throughout the various phases of the community organizing effort. Process or formative evaluations assist the project group in reassessing strategies that have worked and those that have experienced difficulty. Steps are retraced and programs are modified, expanded, or abandoned. At some point, usually near the end of the project, the organization formally assesses what has been learned and determines future directions. Results from the various types of evaluations outlined in Chapter 6 will be helpful in this reassessment period.

Key Elements

1. Update the community analysis. Updating the community analysis and profile involves looking for changes that have occurred in leadership, resources, and organizational relationships in the community. Key community members, opinion leaders, and organizations in a community will change over time. Reviewing these changes may point to a need for new collaborators and for efforts to recruit new board and task force members. Additional organizations may need representation if programs are to be continued. For example, the City Parks and Recreation Office in one community became more active at the end of a demonstration project as it took on responsibility to incorporate more physical activity campaigns into its regularly scheduled agenda of events.

2. Assess effectiveness of intervention programs. The project will most likely be using some type of formal evaluation plan as the basis for examining the success of its intervention efforts. An evaluation plan that includes ongoing monitoring of programs and activities can make possible periodic reviews of the status and progress of each activity. Monitoring involves establishing appropriate record-keeping systems that collect data for analysis and summary. Community groups may need to contract for research expertise in conducting evaluations; local universities and colleges may be willing to assist in such efforts.

A variety of quantitative and qualitative indicators of success can be evaluated. Awareness, participation, support, attendance, and behavior change are examples of quantitative indicators. Qualitative indicators include retention of staff and volunteers, levels of decision making by citizen groups, and feedback and involvement from participants and sponsoring agencies.

Programs are intended to change behaviors and norms and to become institutionalized in the community. Existing organizations may become sponsors or "owners" of specific programs. Some programs may need new sponsors, which will require a longer development period. Other programs may be significantly changed by new sponsors. Some programs will be evaluated as ineffective and will be discarded or modified. Not all programs should be continued indefinitely.

3. Summarize results and chart future directions. Project continuation is partially dependent on maintaining high visibility in the community through effective communication with and further diffusion among key groups within the community. These include leaders, program participants, media representatives, potential support sources, and other influential organizations. Oral and/or written reports can provide information to the community. Simple, concise charts and graphs can communicate results effectively. The process of planning future directions is often a formal one that includes revising and rewriting goals and objectives to reflect the updated community analysis and program evaluations. Some community boards may consider the need for a marketing survey or analysis to determine directions further. Developing a strategy for continued collaboration and networking should be emphasized. Seeking new sources of funding may be required as part of the continuation effort. These efforts toward durability of the project are discussed in detail in Chapter 7.

Overall Challenges to Community Organization in the Future: Concluding Remarks

Citizen participation in organized community groups is a common and expected human norm. Nonetheless, there are barriers to participation that may vary by social context, country, or culture. Pilisuk, McCallister, and Rothman (1996) identified six modern conditions that have changed the context for community organizing. They are the fragmentation of the supportive capacities of communities, that local problems are often manifestations of global problems, the concentration of transnational power, the inaccessibility of information about power in society, the centralized domination of symbols of legitimacy, and the disempowering effects of the mass media. Each of these conditions works against the ability to achieve social change. Nonetheless, the number of grassroots groups has grown internationally, with environmental issues often serving as a catalyst (Pilisuk et al., 1996). In those areas where social reform is most needed, there is almost certain to arise some form of grassroots organizing. It is rare for people with social power to change society radically. Social movements invariably start with grassroots organizing.

Community organization for health can be influenced by the quality of and access to the health system. In those countries where health insurance is universal and services reasonably accessible, there is less pressure for community groups to form to advocate for health services or programs. Countries with a history of substantial government involvement in health planning and prevention programs, such as Australia, have less activism for health service issues than in countries where private health insurance models predominate (such as the United States). A tradition of volunteerism also facilitates participation in voluntary organizations. In countries without such traditions, citizens may expect payment of some kind for services rendered, particularly in areas where governments historically have provided public services, such as health services in Australia. More recently, where health budgets have been reduced in real terms due to the increased cost of health care, greater citizen action has resulted as a consequence of greater perceived need.

As community health promotion programs have proliferated and expanded nationally and internationally, a common set of essential planning and organizing tasks has emerged from these community mobilization and implementation experiences. Programs in dissimilar locales and with different goals encounter common concerns that must be anticipated and planned for. Based on these many community health demonstration projects, the most common issues that arise include (a) selecting community representatives, (b) establishing effective partnerships, (c) achieving mission clarity and program boundaries, (d) identification of resistance, (e) establishing evaluation and tracking mechanisms, (f) successfully managing and reinforcing volunteer involvement, (g) conducting ongoing training and skills development, (h) recruiting field staff with appropriate competencies and experience, and (i) securing resources for maintenance and durability of effort.

Lessons Learned From Project Northland

Community Organization in Rural Communities

SARA VEBLEN-MORTENSON

CHRIS RISSEL

CHERYL L. PERRY

JEAN FORSTER

MARK WOLFSON

JOHN R. FINNEGAN Jr.

This case study focuses on the lessons learned in the initial years of the community intervention component of Project Northland Phase I (1991-1994), a communitywide research project designed to prevent or reduce alcohol use among young adolescents in rural northeastern Minnesota. Also described are recent developments from Phase II (1995-1999), which introduced community social action teams to reduce the commercial and social availability of alcohol to underage youth. The teams initiated strategies to change community norms and practices around underage drinking as well as to reduce underage access to alcohol in the intervention communities.

The primary lessons learned during Phase I were that (a) early citizen perception of the project as a *student-focused* project facilitated community acceptance but also slowed attempts to change local alcohol ordinances and policies, (b) up to 1 year was needed for community needs assessments and local coordinator and task force member training, (c) local paid coordinators required great tact to avoid being socially isolated by other community members and (d) local power dynamics in rural areas differ from those in an urban setting. Each of these lessons is discussed in detail later.

Description of Project Northland

Project Northland is a communitywide research program to prevent young adolescent alcohol use. The project was designed by faculty in the Division of Epidemiology, School of Public Health at the University of Minnesota to test the efficacy of a multilevel, multiyear intervention program for youth (Perry, Williams, Forster, et al., 1993). It is the first such trial that has randomized school districts and adjoining communities to an intervention condition, specifically targeted young adolescent alcohol use, and used a multilevel intervention program. It was anticipated that this multilevel program would change parent-child communication about alcohol use, the functional meanings of alcohol use for young people, the student's self-efficacy to resist alcohol, peer influence to drink, alcohol use norms, and students' perceptions of and actual ease of access to alcohol in their communities (Perry, Williams, Veblen-Mortenson, et al., 1996).

Project Northland, conducted in northeast Minnesota, involves mostly rural, lower-middle-class to middle-class communities. The population of the six participating counties is 235,000, and residents are primarily of European ethnic backgrounds. This area of Minnesota rates at the top in terms of alcohol-related problems in the state (National Institute on Alcohol Abuse and Alcoholism, 1994).

The intervention programs were implemented in the 14 randomly assigned intervention school districts, with adolescents in the class of 1998 during their 6th, 7th, and 8th grades and in the intervention communities as a whole during the same period (1991-1994). Young people were exposed to classroom, school, peer, family, and communitywide programs on alcohol use. This multicomponent intervention focuses on the identified etiological psychosocial risk factors for adolescent alcohol use (Klepp, Perry, & Jacobs, 1991; Perry & Kelder, 1992a, 1992b). These factors are targeted in three ways: through school-based interventions designed to increase peer pressure resistance and social competence skills, through home-based programming to provide parental support and encourage positive modeling, and through communitywide interventions designed to change the larger social environment (Perry, Williams, Forster, et al., 1993). The communitywide interventions complement and support the work being done in the schools and with parents. Much of the specific school and parent-focused intervention activities is based on social cognitive theory (Bandura, 1977, 1986). The communitywide components of Project Northland are based on community organization theory. The emphasis of this case study focuses on the communitywide components.

Community Organization Theory

Underpinning Project Northland's first phase of community intervention is the five-stage model of community organization for health promotion elaborated by Bracht, Kingsbury, and Rissel (chapter 4). Application of the model to Project Northland is shown in Table CI4.1. This model has been applied to a number of community-based demonstration projects.

STAGE 1: COMMUNITY ANALYSIS

The community analysis was conducted to understand how the education communities function at a public level, to collect baseline data, and to identify key people to involve in the project (Finnegan, Bracht, & Viswanath, 1989). The primary tool used for this analysis was a community leader survey. The purpose of this survey was to collect data that characterized power and leadership structures in each town, to assess leaders' views of adolescent alcohol access restriction policies, to assess community expectations about underage drinking, and to identify key community leaders and activists who might join the community task forces. Selection criteria were developed for the 28 communities that participated in the survey. In each community, five leaders were surveyed, including the mayor, police chief (or local law enforcement officer), chair of the local Chamber of Commerce or business association, the local newspaper editor (weekly or daily), and the senior education official residing in the community (usually a principal) (Perry, Williams, Forster, et al., 1993).

STAGE 2: DESIGN AND INITIATION

The principle mechanism for initiating community efforts to prevent or reduce adolescent alcohol use in Project Northland is community task forces. Local project coordinators recruited adults in the community to participate in a Project Northland task force. Coordinators were asked to contact key leaders across a range of sectors within the community (coordinators had access to the results from the community analysis survey mentioned above). When a substantial number of community members had been recruited, the first task force member training session was held.

STAGE 3: IMPLEMENTATION

An attempt was made during this stage to promote and support the philosophy of partnership and collaboration central to the principles of effective participation in community organization (Bracht & Tsouros, 1990) and yet also provide direction and guidance to the task forces. A "menu" of community strategies for preventing alcohol use among young teens was developed for task force members (see Table CI4.2). This menu provided examples of community policy options and prevention strategies to limit alcohol access to young teens in four major areas: (a) voluntary efforts and community education, (b) enforcement of existing laws, (c) the adoption of local ordinances and administrative policies, and (d) institutional policies. This menu was not exhaustive but provided examples of the range of local intervention strategies that might influence social or legal availability of alcohol for young people. These options also included measures designed to influence community norms and attitudes about the appropriate role of alcohol vis-à-vis youth. This list also represents a range in terms of expected political

TABLE CI4.1 Five-Stage Model of Community Organization for Health Promotion[a] and
Its Application in Project Northland

Theoretical Model	Project Northland Activities
Stage 1: Community analysis	
Define the community	14 education and 10 control communities randomly selected in northeastern Minnesota
Collect data	Baseline data collected on adolescent alcohol use, access to alcohol assessed through merchant and alcohol purchase survey and parent survey
Assess community capacity	Community leadership survey, archival data
Synthesize data and set priorities	The project focus is on the prevention of alcohol use by young adolescents
Stage 2: Design and initiation	
Select a local organizer or coordinator	Field staff were employed who reside in education communities and have experience working in schools and communities
Choose an organization structure	Community task force approach adopted
Identify, select, and recruit organization members	Recruitment of task force members from leadership list and from social and professional networks of local coordinators
Define the organizations' goals	Project goal of prevention of alcohol use by young adolescents is emphasized; task force develops mission statement, goals, and objectives
Clarify staff roles and responsibilities	Individual task forces develop statement of task force membership roles and responsibilities
Provide training and recognition	Two major training events occurred where all task force members were invited, and university staff attended various local meetings

opposition and amount of prior experience in other communities with these measures. In the
first year of the intervention, the task forces were asked to choose three goals from the menu to
pursue.

STAGE 4: MAINTENANCE

During the first phase of Project Northland, the task forces were in operation for
approximately 24 months. A survey of all 88 adult task force members at 6 months, as part of
routine process evaluation, revealed general satisfaction with the groups and agreement with
their direction (Rissel, Finnegan, Wolfson, & Perry, 1995). A number of community programs
and policies were implemented. The task forces were involved in the passage of five alcohol-
related city ordinances and three city resolutions. Ordinances that have been passed include the
establishment of responsible beverage server training in four communities, an ordinance stating

TABLE CI4.1 Continued

Theoretical Model	Project Northland Activities
Stage 3: Implementation	
Generate broad citizen participation	Parents and community members were recruited to assist with the organization and implementation of alcohol-free recreational activities for adolescents
Develop a sequential work plan	All task forces were asked to generate an annual plan of activities
Use comprehensive, integrated strategies	Where possible, task force activities reinforced school-based and parent involvement activities
Integrate community values into program	All Project Northland activities are sensitive to the local culture, with local coordinators and task force members advising on acceptability
Stage 4: Program maintenance and consolidation	
Integrate intervention activities into community networks	Presentations were given throughout community groups and organizations; Speakers Kit' was developed for task forces as a resource guide for presentations about the aims of Project Northland
Establish a positive organizational culture	Regular productive meetings, networking with other groups with related missions and activities
Establish an ongoing recruitment plan	Expanded recruitment planned to include residents who have lived all their lives in the area
Disseminate results	Ongoing feedback to community of results of research activity
Stage 5: Dissemination or reassessment	
Update the community analysis	Community leader survey
Assess effectiveness of interventions	Outcomes data reviewed
Chart future directions and modifications	Direct action model adopted
Summarize and disseminate results	Action teams receive Ph I data reports

a. Bracht and Kingsbury (1990).

certain conditions for the renewal and granting of liquor licenses, and requirements for liquor establishment closing hours. Resolutions passed were in regard to (a) identifying underage drinking in the Grand Rapids/Itasca County area as unacceptable behavior and supporting the laws that already exist and (b) establishment of a designated beer-selling and drinking area at public events in another community. Another action that was taken was the blocking of a resolution to authorize a 10 a.m., as opposed to a 12 p.m., bar service hour on Sundays for bars in one community.

Other activities that task forces have undertaken include letter writing campaigns, community education via health fairs and submission of news articles in the local paper, encouraging the posting of and actively distributing merchant display materials that discourage

TABLE CI4.2 Community Policy "Menu" of Interventions to Reduce Alcohol Access
              to Teenagers

Voluntary efforts, community education
- Provide alcohol-free recreational events and gathering places
- Encourage news reporting of alcohol-related problems and crashes
- Establish an alcohol awareness week with appropriate community activities
- Educate merchants about alcohol problems, strategies to reduce underage sales
- Work with youth-oriented adult groups to increase awareness, generate support for policy approaches
- Publicize server liability laws
- Call public attention to advertisements that appeal to youth
- Establish speakers' bureaus

Enforcement of existing laws
- Encourage enforcement of:
- minimum-age-of-sale laws
- laws against alcohol use in public places
- laws against adults providing alcohol to youth

Local ordinances, administrative policies
- Require training and certification of alcohol sellers and servers
- Restrict alcohol sales at sporting, music, and other public events
- Restrict number, type, and location of alcohol outlets, using zoning ordinances
- Restrict alcohol advertising on billboards at public events, on public property
- Eliminate alcohol industry and outlet sponsorship of local events
- Require public hearings for new and renewal liquor licenses
- Require beer kegs to be tagged with purchaser's name and address

Institutional policies
- Eliminate alcohol at any school functions
- Develop sanctions for alcohol users at nonschool events
- Increase enforcement of school-based policies
- Provide model alcohol polices for recreational settings

---

alcohol sales to minors, sponsorship of speakers for parent and young teenagers' groups, community survey to assess community opinions related to young adolescent alcohol use, and sponsoring activities in school facilities for young teens on weekends. Collaboration with other community and parent groups to sponsor and initiate alcohol-free activities and the development and implementation of alternative activities for young teens has been a priority for most of the task forces. One particularly innovative strategy was the initiation of a "Gold Card" program in five school districts. This involves local community businesses offering teenage nonusers of alcohol a discount.

Lessons Learned During Stages 1 Through 4

After the first 2 years of supporting active task forces and 3 years of experience working with the local Project Northland coordinators, several lessons about community organization in rural settings have been learned. Discussions of the consequences of these observations are presented, and then recommendations are made based on the Project Northland experiences.

The observations and insights offered below are largely those from project staff who have worked closely with the coordinators and task forces. These reflections highlight potential problem areas and issues that may require particular attention in rural communities.

IDENTIFICATION OF PROJECT NORTHLAND AS A
SCHOOL-BASED PROGRAM FOR YOUNG ADOLESCENTS

Although Project Northland was conceived of as a communitywide program, intervention was initiated primarily in the schools. From the outset, liaison has been between the University of Minnesota and representatives in the school districts. The majority of the projects' resources are directed toward the student cohort, with the evaluation designed to detect changes in student behavior resulting from school curriculum-based interventions. The first public activity of Project Northland was a classroom-based intervention in the 6th grade called the Slick Tracy Home Team program. This six-session, 6-week classroom and home-based alcohol use prevention program was designed for 6th-grade students and their parents, who could use it to begin the process of learning and communicating about alcohol use issues. The communitywide activities of Project Northland supplement the work in the schools.

In at least 14 of the 20 intervention communities involved in the project, the school is the economic and social center of the community. Generally, much community activity is initiated by the schools, and many community leaders have strong associations with the schools. Early identification of Project Northland with the schools directly influenced community members' perceptions of the task forces and how task force members perceived their roles. Task force members perceived their role to be to assist in the provision of alternative (to alcohol) activities for teenagers and were often reluctant to consider working on policy options that would not directly affect adolescents or that seemed to fall outside of the schools' jurisdiction, such as advocating for restrictions on the consumption of alcohol by adults in public places.

Project Northland was initially seen to be working toward preventing alcohol use for young adolescents and not directed at adult use. This image was actively promoted in the media to diffuse the sensitive nature of the issue. This project image was nonthreatening to adults and led to widespread acceptance and support of the program. Gradually, this acceptance broadened to include efforts to change adult alcohol norms whenever those norms could be seen to affect adolescent alcohol use.

Initial identification of Project Northland with the schools and having a focus on adolescent alcohol use meant early positive acceptance of the program by the community. Although this slowed efforts by university staff and local coordinators to broaden the focus of the task forces to affect community alcohol policies, the high level of community acceptance of the program may have been necessary for the community policy initiatives to be accepted. The focus on young adolescent alcohol use helped Project Northland avoid potentially damaging controversy and negative reaction. Other practitioners should take particular care to consider the type of program image they are presenting to the community. Given the deeply rooted social, cultural, and historical associations with alcohol in this region, we felt that treading lightly on adult alcohol use and being positively identified with the school would allow the community organization work to be initiated in a more effective manner. Strong identification with the schools made work with the school staff easier but perhaps slowed broader efforts in the community.

FUNDING TIME FRAMES VERSUS COMMUNITY TIME FRAMES

The objectives of Project Northland are to prevent or delay the onset of alcohol use by adolescents. Such an ambitious goal requires time, particularly in an area historically noted for its heavy alcohol use. In an attempt to speed up this process, university-based Project Northland researchers collected the needs assessment data not only from leaders in the intervention communities but also from alcohol merchants and from sociodemographic data about the communities (Perry, Williams, Forster, et al., 1993).

Once these data were collected, field staff were employed. Field staff were hired in October 1991, and the first task force training session took place in April 1992. During this time, the field staff were trained and had to familiarize themselves with their job and community. The first year's school intervention program was implemented, and, at the same time, field staff were expected to recruit community members for the task forces.

Field staff were given suggestions about recruitment. These included that multiple sectors of the community be represented on the task force (such as churches, businesses, schools, government, and social services), as well as "community influentials" (people and organizations with influence in the community) in different sectors. The task forces were also presented with local summaries of the needs assessment data. It was thought that by providing relevant data immediately to the task force members, they would be able to move more quickly into their community work.

A consequence of attempting to speed up the needs assessment process by having university-based staff perform this work was that the field staff and task force members were not actively involved in the definition of the problem. They had not yet come to understand the parameters of adolescent alcohol use through their own needs assessment efforts, and they were simply not ready to tackle potentially controversial and difficult community alcohol policy issues. Insufficient time was allowed for the task forces to fully understand the problem they were dealing with and to "own" the problem. Trust had not yet developed, either of other task force members or by the task force's community.

The time frame for community projects should allow adequate time for field staff and community task force members to learn the dimensions of the problem they are planning to tackle and so understand for themselves the strategies that are most appropriate in their circumstances. With Project Northland, this process did not occur until approximately 8 to 12 months after the first task force training session.

UNDERSTANDING POLICY AND POLICY ADVOCACY

It was envisaged that the task forces would be strong advocates for community policies and ordinances that reduce access to alcohol by adolescents and reduce social support of alcohol use by adolescents. The concept of *policy* (which we defined as "rules or principles that communities formally use to say what is okay to do and what is not okay to do") and the thought of working toward new policies was, somewhat unexpectedly, not enthusiastically embraced by the field staff and task forces. In fact, there was considerable resistance to suggestions that task force efforts be directed towards policy change. Policy initiatives seemed distal and irrelevant to many task force members and local coordinators who, at first, found it difficult to see what effects policy would have on adolescent alcohol use, particularly use by a young cohort of 6th, 7th, and 8th graders. For example, several of the policy recommendations pertained to the commercial availability of alcohol to minors—through sales at bars or liquor stores. Many task force members, as well as project field staff, found it difficult to see the relationship between (for example) a requirement that bar servers receive training ("Responsible Beverage Service") and alcohol use by 6th or 7th graders. Imagined conflict arising from university staff suggestions that new policies were necessary also generated resistance. There was a general lack of experience working with policies that contributed to the threatening aspects of policy work.

Consequently, for the first year, few of the task force activities were directed at changes in community alcohol policy, at least compared to university expectations. Those policies that were pursued were typically nonthreatening to alcohol merchants or other influential segments of the community who might be likely to oppose more vigorous measures. Suggestions were made about new alcohol policies, typically when it seemed "safe."

Inexperience in working at the policy level by task force members and university staff resulted in overly high expectations about changing and/or enforcing policies. Early clarification of what policy is and the process of changing or implementing policies might have reduced resistance to working with policies. Specific early training in strategies to deal with conflict (real or imagined) and in demystifying the political process of establishing policies might also have helped overcome initial resistance.

Moreover, providing specific community organizing training in such areas as mapping the power structure of the community (through one-on-one interviews with community members) and developing a power base for advocacy efforts would have put field staff in a better position to take on potentially conflictual issues. However, these efforts are time consuming and therefore costly. Ongoing research should assess the long-term effectiveness of these approaches (Wagenaar & Perry, 1994).

BARRIERS TO RISK TAKING BY LOCAL COORDINATORS

One aspect of the reluctance of task forces to move forward on policy issues has been the role of the local Project Northland field coordinators. The coordinators, who all live in or near the communities with which they are working, all expressed the desire for caution in how they proceeded in developing Project Northland policy suggestions. As in many rural communities, there is often general resistance to change and local pressure to maintain the status quo (Merry, 1984). The local coordinators walk a fine line between keeping the peace and advancing Project Northland's objectives.

The perception that others might consider the coordinators as dissidents or prohibitionists meant that coordinators and task force members were extremely careful in the selection of task force activities. One coordinator openly expressed this fear by wondering if he would be "tarred and feathered and run of town" as a result of involvement in Project Northland.

These fears were dealt with in Project Northland in a number of ways. The focus on young adolescents was consistently and repeatedly emphasized. Policy options that were first addressed by task forces focused on enforcing existing policies (illegal to provide alcohol to those under 21) and requiring training and certification of alcohol sellers and servers. More difficult policy options, such as restricting alcohol availability at public events, were not addressed until the coordinators felt more comfortable raising them in the community. University faculty and staff had to revise ambitious timeframes and targets for what policies could be implemented.

THE FOCUS OF FIELD COORDINATOR EFFORTS

As the coordinators were primarily school-based, their time was divided between supporting the school curricula and the task forces. The concrete and tangible tasks and rewards of implementing well-defined school-related activities were clearly preferred by many of the coordinators to the nebulous activities of policy advocacy and the resistance and less positive feedback from the task forces. As many of the coordinators were employed on a part-time basis, their time was thinly spread.

Initiating and maintaining communitywide activities requires considerable time and energy. Coordinators were given the task of coordinating and implementing school-based, parent, and peer activities, as well as organizing communitywide activities with task forces in 20 to 30 hours per week. Staff need appropriate funding and time to carry out all of the activities necessary to make a communitywide effort successful.

GENDER ROLES

Despite equal employment and antidiscrimination legislation, gender differences were evident in the rural areas covered by Project Northland. A Project Northland survey of positional leaders (e.g., mayors, police chiefs, editors, school principals, business leaders) revealed that the leaders were predominately male. Females are not as frequently part of the formal power network. Anecdotal stories from the coordinators and task force members reveal that much of the local business and government work is done within these essentially male informal networks. It should be noted that many of the Project Northland communities were founded as iron mining towns, which were traditionally male dominated.

The male networks in northeastern Minnesota do not stop women from occupying positions of government or power. However, women may not have the same type of informal access to those in power and are often excluded from these networks. Consequently, male coordinators may feel they have more to lose (i.e., exclusion from informal networks that they are a part of) by attempting to implement controversial alcohol policies than female coordinators. Female coordinators have reported having to work more "delicately" with men in authority to have their or their task forces' perspective treated seriously. This was compounded by the high proportion of women (69%) on the task forces (Rissel et al., 1995). The need for tact is not uncommon among women attempting to assume positions of power in a traditionally patriarchal society (Soh, 1993). Sensitivity to the dynamics of power and gender was required by all Project Northland staff. University staff need to work within these constraints and be sensitive to the realities of local communities.

RURAL VERSUS URBAN DYNAMICS OF POWER

A primary difference between the rural and urban context for community organization work is the degree of anonymity communities afford. In an urban context, it is more likely that an activist will not personally know the officials who are being lobbied. Confrontational tactics and strategies may have fewer interpersonal risks. In a rural context, where community members know each other well, such conflict-generating strategies may not be as successful. Project Northland coordinators report that conflict certainly exists but is dangerous in the sense that the continued viability of a "player" (in political contests) may be threatened.

Because the coordinators and task force members must continue to live in the communities where they are working, a strong feeling of caution is evident when considering potentially conflict-generating strategies to implement community alcohol policies. A clear preference for strategies that are more consensual exists.

In addition, the fact that coordinators were not explicitly encouraged to map the power structure of their communities meant that they sometimes lacked the information needed to develop effective political strategies in pursuing policy change. Moreover, task force recruitment was not as effective as it might have been. Project coordinators often recruited community members who were known to them (Rissel et al., 1995) and, also, who often had experience mainly in the educational arena. Thus, coordinators often lacked a team within which effective policy advocacy strategies could be planned and implemented.

Learning who the key people in the Project Northland intervention communities are has been important. The leadership survey was a key component in identifying leaders who were important in a number of different sectors. These people were invited to participate in the task forces, and 30% of the identified leaders did attend task force meetings. However, those people who are considered influential tend also to be very busy, and their attendance at task force meetings has not always been consistent. Attrition of these key players requires an on-going search for new members or ways to involve key leaders.

In summary, Project Northland staff have been careful to avoid potential conflict and controversy (by focusing on young adolescent alcohol use) and initially to support "safer" task force strategies of promoting responsible beverage service, providing alternative activities for teenagers, and structuring incentives for young people to remain alcohol free. It was important to invite influential community leaders to join the community task forces, and it has been important that field coordinators realized that continual recruitment is necessary. The association of key leaders with the task forces may be all that can be expected, and their support may be a sufficient contribution. Thus, a major Project Northland strategy has been to continually create linkages between key sectors within the community: schools, business, church, parents, teens, the public health community.

Stage 5: Community Intervention
Reassessment and Adjustments

Although Project Northland had success in delaying onset and reducing the prevalence of alcohol use as well as changing key psychosocial factors at the end of the first phase of the research (1991-1994) (Perry, Williams, Veblen-Mortenson, et al., 1996), the larger social environment was less likely to be affected, including actual access to alcohol and perceptions of teens' ability to obtain alcohol in the community (Perry, Williams, Veblen-Mortenson, et al., 1996). Reassessment of the community intervention component for Phase II of Project Northland was based on Phase I data, lessons learned from the community intervention during Phase I, and on knowledge of prior research and experience (Forster et al., in press; Wagenaar & Perry, 1994). Prior research suggests that the community organization model adopted during Phase II would be potentially powerful in affecting community norms related to adolescents' alcohol use and in increasing community efficacy to take action to reduce alcohol use among adolescents.

Given the outcomes of the first phase of the project (Perry, Williams, Veblen-Mortenson, et al., 1996), it was clear that the intervention focus during Phase II (1995-1998) needed to shift from a primary focus on what are called "demand factors," or reducing teens' desire to drink alcohol through education, development of skills for refusing alcohol, communication with parents and peers, and participation in positive, alcohol-free activities, to more of a focus on "supply factors," or reducing the availability of alcohol by targeting community-level factors that influence underage drinking. This shift meant that although intervention strategies during the second phase still incorporated demand factors, given the comprehensive nature of the intervention, more of an emphasis was given to targeting supply factors.

Of the five intervention components implemented during Phase II—community action teams, youth action teams, school prevention programs, parent involvement and education, and media—the community action teams were formed to address supply factors by initiating prevention activities to reduce the commercial and social availability of alcohol to underage youth. The newly developed action teams were similar to task forces in that they served as the mechanism for initiating community efforts. However, a different model using "direct action" community organizing was adopted to guide the action teams' development and implementation during Phase II.

A direct action community organizing model was used to promote and create policy change at the local level with endeavors not related specifically to public health. It sought to change community policies and practices by mobilizing a large proportion of the community, who used their collective power to alter the locus of decision making and resource distribution (Hanna & Robinson, 1994). It was clear that a focus on implementing environmental prevention strategies, primarily through policy changes, would call for more active and widespread community acceptance and participation.

This model has also been used in previous public health research in increasing participation, ownership, control, and capacity of individuals and communities to engage institutions and community members in defining problems and designing public health action strategies in tobacco use prevention that affected adolescent health outcomes (ASSIST Working Group on Durability, 1996; Blaine et al., 1997; Forster et al., in press).

The community organizing social action process consisted of four stages: (a) training on direct action community organizing, (b) extensive interviews ($N = 100$ [average, with fewer in the smallest communities] within each community with populations ranging from 250 to 8,000) conducted by the community organizers within all sectors of the community to determine citizens' motivation and self-interest for action, (c) recruitment and formation of a core action team of 5 to 12 community members to lead the effort in their communities, and (d) implementation of alcohol-related ordinances, policies, and practices to change community norms and practices regarding underage drinking and to reduce underage access to alcohol.

The community organizing training provided the organizers with the framework to implement the components of the model and a foundation of information and skills that would better prepare them to deal with the issues that arose in Phase I. The training included (a) a better understanding of the power structures within organizers' communities so that they could more effectively obtain the assistance of those individuals or groups to implement appropriate prevention initiatives, (b) a framework for mobilizing organizers' communities to gain a groundswell of support for limiting youth access to alcohol, (c) more knowledge of policy content and a process for implementing policy within organizers' communities, and (d) a model for more effectively dealing with conflict in the communities as policy options were adopted and implemented.

The training prepared the organizers to formulate action teams that would build on previous task force activity yet attempt to implement prevention activities with more of a policy orientation and a larger base of citizen participation.

Eleven Project Northland community action teams, representing 14 communities, have been working for the past 2 years to build community support for and to implement policies, ordinances, and practices that reduce youth access to alcohol. The results from Phase II of the community intervention will be reported when the project reaches its conclusion.

In summary, the lessons learned from the first phase of Project Northland's community intervention provide insight to the challenges that public health practitioners and community members may face when establishing policies and practices to prevent and reduce underage drinking in rural areas. The addition of social action initiatives in Phase II was designed to more strategically target community level factors and mobilize whole communities for prevention.

It is clear from over a decade of public health research that the best way to achieve and sustain prevention is to target both individuals and their environments (Gardner, Green, & Marcus, 1994) and that demand and supply factors must be targeted simultaneously. The complement of individual and environmental level changes, accompanied by widespread community acceptance and support of these prevention initiatives, may be the key to effective and long-lasting alcohol prevention efforts.

5

Mass Media and Health Promotion

Lessons Learned, With Implications for Public Health Campaigns

JOHN R. FINNEGAN JR.

K. VISWANATH

Since before the development of the mass media, communication campaigns have been regarded as central in educating and persuading the public to take action to ameliorate disease and promote health. One of the first such efforts on the North American continent occurred in the 1750s in Boston. The Rev. Cotton Mather used the power of the pulpit, the pamphlet, and colonial newspapers to persuade the city's residents to seek vaccination against smallpox, which periodically ravaged the population (Paisley, 1981). Although Mather's effort was not free of opposition, it established the organized campaign as the preferred vehicle in America to promote population health through voluntary adoption of behavior change. This pattern has continued to the present day but in the context of a global, interconnected media and public health environment that Mather could scarcely have envisioned some 240 years ago.

In the past 20 years especially, a great deal has been learned about public health campaigns and the roles of the mass media in successful and not-so-successful efforts to prevent disease and to promote health. This chapter reviews these lessons, learned from recent experience, and translates them into practical strategies to guide community health campaign planners and public health advocates. Specifically, we review recent thought about the roles and functions of the mass media in the context of a dramatically changing media environment, how these relate to public health and community-based campaign theory, and, finally, the successes and pitfalls public health advocates face in using the mass media to effect change in population health.

Media Roles

Although movable type made possible the widespread dissemination of the printed word beginning in the mid-15th century, it was not until the 17th century that newspapers, the first public medium, emerged in Britain, Europe, and the Americas. However, it was not until 1833 that the first mass circulation newspapers capable of reaching most if not all of the population emerged in the United States (Emery & Emery, 1996). Thus the "mass media" that we take for granted today are a relatively recent phenomenon in human history, about 165 years old. The mid-19th century also witnessed the emergence of the first electronic medium, the telegraph, in 1844. For the first time, communication was possible at speeds far exceeding the fastest form of transportation.

Technologic development of the mass media has continued in the 20th century at a breakneck pace to create the complex, global media infrastructure with which we are familiar today. But equally as important as the technology that produced the mass media, has been the media's evolution as powerful institutions, with significant social, political, and economic impact on communities and nations. Communication theorists have defined this influence in four crucial media roles: (a) surveillance and interpretation of the environment, (b) entertainment, (c) advertising, and (d) transmission of a social and cultural heritage (Lasswell, 1948). The mass media's primary purpose is not the same as public health, but these roles form the basis of the media's capacity to propel (or retard) the goals of public health. How well the media function on behalf of public health goals is significantly influenced by how well the media are engaged by the field of public health itself.

Media Uses

Communication theorists note the importance of the mass media in defining significant issues and information for the public, communities, and societies. This is the *agenda-setting* function by which the media confer importance and legitimacy on issues, by devoting attention to them (McCombs, 1992; McCombs & Shaw, 1977, 1993). This powerful function is embodied in surveys that show a strong relationship between what the public believes are important issues and issues that the media actually report. However, the media not only define what is important but also provide frameworks within which to interpret or understand information about the issues (Clarke, 1991). That is, news stories provide "frames" within which we interpret issues and events in some ways but not others.

The media do not carry out these functions autonomously. What the media report in the first place, and how they report is strongly influenced by other institutions such as government, public and private organizations, advocacy groups, and so on. Media research tells us that the activity of these news sources is key in defining for the media which issues are important and the way in which the issues are framed (Hilgartner & Bosk, 1988; Kosicki, 1993; Roshco, 1975; Sigal, 1987;

Tuchman, 1978). This aspect of the media's agenda-setting function is supported by studies that demonstrate that much, if not most, "news" may be traced to specific sources representing various institutions and groups (Shoemaker, 1991).

This media function is also key in community-based health promotion. Media are important to achieving the goals of public health, first, because they raise the public profile of issues in bringing them to the attention of the community. Second, they confer importance and legitimacy to the issues as relevant to community concerns. Third, they provide frameworks of meaning within which to understand issues (e.g., risk, effective preventive actions, behavioral norms, the need for public policy, and so on). Fourth, the media are capable of widespread public dissemination of, and exposure to, public health information.

Some Lessons Learned and Practical Implications

Some of the important lessons learned about the use of mass media in the past 20 years of community-based public health campaigns include

1. *Planning is key to the effective engagement of the mass media in public health campaigns.*

Public health advocates have usually planned campaigns with media components using two approaches: social marketing and media advocacy. Social marketing is a planning framework developed in the early 1970s, wherein the object is the promotion of ideas, norms, and behavior change rather than the commercial goal of selling goods and services (Kotler & Roberto, 1989). It establishes a process requiring clarity and specificity in setting campaign objectives, in conducting formative evaluation to delineate target audiences, effective message and program elements, and channels with the influence and reach to affect target audiences. Formative research is central to the process, as is clarifying community barriers and opportunities to reaching specified objectives. Social marketing may be used whether the objective is to influence individual behavior change or in advocating change in public policy (Lefebvre, 1992). In either case, the process results in a clear plan integrating intervention components that include the mass media and specifying the timing, delivery, and evaluation of results in communities.

Media advocacy uses mass media and community organizing strategies specifically to advance a social or public policy initiative (Jernigan & Wright, 1996; Wallack, Dorfman, Jernigan, & Themba, 1993). Population behavior change is certainly the outcome envisioned in both approaches, but media advocacy seeks such change specifically through policy rather than direct appeals for voluntary behavior change by specific target audiences, which is more common in public health applications of social marketing. Media advocacy is more explicit about using the power and influence of the mass media's agenda-setting functions to effect social and public policy change. Yet both approaches are similar in their use of careful planning involving the mass media.

2. *Mass media may be engaged in public health campaigns at different levels of involvement.*

At the most basic level, community public health campaigns may seek to engage the media in providing occasional publicity through news stories, columns, or the kind of community bulletin board that frequently appears in newspapers or on the radio or other media. More often, they seek sustained media interest in the campaign. This requires long-term thinking about campaign objectives and relating these to media "news values" for stories that are new, dramatic, important, include conflict or have strong human interest angles. For example, media advocacy strategies often emphasize sustaining media interest in an issue through the use of "creative epidemiology," which seeks to put a human face on the dry statistics of risk through the use of dramatic metaphors (Wallack et al., 1993). Social marketing, too, emphasizes the production of messages with special relevance and interest for prospective target groups.

Media interest may also be sustained in the long term by seeking to form partnerships with the media in achieving campaign goals. This is a strategy in which the media become a major stakeholder in the campaign along with other community groups and interests and actively participate in campaign planning and implementation. This was a strategy that worked effectively for the Stanford Heart Disease Prevention Project (SHDPP) in the 1970s and 1980s. More recently, the media have become deeply involved in public service campaigns, including public health, as part of a media movement called "Civic Journalism" or the "New Public Journalism" (Merritt & Rosen, 1995). Stung by criticism that the media have more negative than positive impact, many media outlets have sought to reconnect with their communities through public service projects.

3. *Engaging the mass media in public health campaigns means in part establishing good working relationships with media "gatekeepers."*

Successful engagement of the mass media on behalf of public health campaigns requires an understanding of community media systems, the culture and habits of media work, and the structure of media organizations. An early step in any public health campaign that seeks to engage the media requires first creating a community "media profile" that describes a community's media system, including print, display, and electronic media as well as public relations, advertising, and other communication agencies and organizations. Several different national media directories available in reference libraries provide a great deal of information about media outlets (e.g., Editor & Publisher Newspaper Directory, Broadcasting and Cable Yearbook, Burelle's Media Directory). This includes general information about media organizations, ownership, and audience "reach" or circulation and also identifies key individuals in media organizations who control access: reporters and editors in the print media and reporters, news directors, and producers in the electronic media. Directories are often cross indexed by community or geographical area to permit easy location of media outlets.

Although campaign planners' interests in the media usually focus on print and electronic media, it may also be helpful to cast the net wider to include public relations, advertising, and other communication firms that work closely with media outlets. Many such agencies offer some pro bono services to community organizations or worthy community causes. In addition, their deep knowledge of, and contacts with, community media may help to shorten the process of making the right media contacts and help public health campaigns to better refine their media strategies.

The media's purposes are not the same as public health's, but it would be incorrect to assume that the media do not share many of the same goals as public health advocates. Media organizations are embedded in communities like other social institutions and are composed of people who want the best for their communities. Moreover, most media outlets are in the business of gathering, processing, and publishing news of interest and relevance to their communities. They cannot successfully function without groups, coalitions, and advocates working with them to identify important issues and information and to help the media bring them to the public's attention.

At one level, engaging media interest on behalf of a community public health campaign means establishing good working relationships with media editors, producers and reporters. This means functioning as a good news source in explaining the goals of the campaign, providing background, and assisting the media in developing interesting and provocative stories for readers and viewers. This will likely involve helping them make contacts in the community for story development as well as being easily available to help them make deadlines and do a thorough job of reporting. In part, this requires the public health advocate to put himself or herself in the editor's or reporter's shoes to think about what is actually "newsworthy." For media like television, there is the added burden of thinking about interesting visuals.

There are a variety of "dos" and "don'ts" in developing and maintaining good relationships with the media, but mainly they are commonsense guidelines based on mutual professional respect (for some further discussion, consult the community education section of the website http:// epihub.epi.umn.edu/REACT).

4. *The mass media can be highly effective in building the community agenda for public policy change on behalf of public health, but media attention alone is seldom sufficient without sustained efforts by empowered community groups and coalitions.*

This is a key conclusion of Jernigan and Wright (1996), who reviewed a number of case studies using media advocacy to influence public policies related to alcohol marketing, access, advertising, and taxation. The authors found that although media attention was critical to the policy-making process, the ability to maintain influence generally requires broad-based community coalitions with a long-range vision and planned strategies to counter potential opposition. Thus community organizing is regarded as central to successful media advocacy strategies.

5. *The mass media's impact as part of community-based campaigns to affect health behavior or policy is considerable but is attenuated by the socioeconomic structure of communities.*

A great deal of communication research has demonstrated that media campaign exposure and effects do not occur equally across all social groups. Campaign researchers have long recognized this, but it was not until the 1970s that this finding was first articulated by Minnesota researchers Donohue, Olien, and Tichenor (1990) as the "Knowledge Gap Hypothesis." They argued that lower socioeconomic status (SES) groups usually benefited less from media campaigns (including public health) than higher SES groups. Although they noted that social conflict, motivational differences, and other factors may at times reduce "gaps" in knowledge, information, and learning between groups, SES differences in these effects are usually present and long lasting. For example, Donohue et al. noted that the impact of media-generated information on public knowledge and opinion is not uniformly distributed among social groups. In examining national polls, they found that the most dramatic increase in beliefs that smoking is a health threat occurred among those with the highest levels of formal education (from about 49% in 1954 to about 92% in 1981). Those with the least formal education (a measure of SES) increased from about 40% in 1954 to about 73% in 1981. The medium-education group increased from about 40% in 1954 to about 84% in 1981. Although each group increased in their beliefs in the dangers of smoking, there were greater differences between the highest education and lowest education groups by 1981 than was true in 1954. The authors have suggested that such knowledge gaps are likely due to the effects of differential exposure and access to mass media and perhaps other deficits of social structural origin, including literacy and the relevance of information.

Finnegan, Viswanath, Kahn, and Hannan (1993) focused on exposure to sources of heart disease prevention information in the MHHP reference communities. They showed that over time (1980-1989), groups with the lowest formal education (less than a high school education) were significantly less likely to report as many sources of heart disease information as those with greater formal education. The same finding was true in examining the diversity of sources as well as newspaper and other print sources reported. However, educational level did not differentiate reporting of television and other electronic media as sources of heart disease information. Viswanath, Finnegan, Hertog, Pirie, and Murray (1994) similarly reported that the diffusion of information about local heart health programs spread differentially among social groups. Less-educated groups became aware of the programs later than groups with more formal education.

Davis, Winkleby, and Farquhar (1995) analyzed heart disease prevention knowledge among different SES groups in cities of the Stanford Heart Disease Prevention Program (SHDPP) from 1980 to 1990. They discovered significant differences and widening gaps in knowledge, with the lowest SES groups benefiting least from the campaigns. Individuals with less than a high school education experienced only modest improvement in their knowledge of heart disease risk factors; those with a college degree or more improved twice as much. These findings remained despite nonsignificantly different (and high) levels of interest in heart disease risk modification across all SES levels.

In a study of SES and smoking, Millar (1996) found that although smoking rates have declined among all groups, they have declined least among lower SES groups. Compared to higher SES groups, lower SES groups also reported fewer sources of information about smoking (including the mass media) and were less likely to report sources of printed information. Lower SES groups also reported encountering fewer smoking restrictions in their daily lives.

The practical realities of SES-based differences in media exposure and impact argue for attention to several strategies, as follows:

- Reaching lower SES groups through influential channels, which may include a mix of media, group, and interpersonal strategies;
- Crafting and testing of media messages, with special attention to values, interest, and relevance affecting lower SES groups;
- Developing messages with special attention to media formats requiring minimal print literacy;
- Engaging lower SES groups directly in the process of planning, developing, and implementing a campaign with mass media components.

6. *Influencing entertainment programming to carry health messages is a less developed but promising strategy for use of mass media in public health campaigns.*

Media content, particularly on television, is mainly entertainment rather than news. News frequently has a more limited appeal, but entertainment appeals to nearly everyone. Entertainment programming has the potential not only to reach a larger audience but to provide health behavior messages in a more palatable, culturally appropriate and interesting format. This was discovered somewhat by accident in Peru in the 1970s through a soap opera entitled *Simplemente Maria* (Singhal, Obregon, & Rogers, 1994; Svenkerud, Rahoi, & Singhal, 1995). The fictional program told the story of a poor young woman who became wealthy by purchasing a sewing machine and training herself as a seamstress. The show caused many poor young Peruvian women to actually emulate the character's strategy in their efforts to overcome their poverty.

Public health advocates and filmmakers realized the potential for such programming also to educate about public health behavior and norms. The technique has been tried with some success in the developing world, including Mexico, Central and South America, India, and Africa, with particular effectiveness among poor, illiterate audiences (Singhal, Rogers, & Brown, 1993; Svenkerud et al., 1995). Although less used in the United States, the strategy has nevertheless met with some success. Most notably, Harvard public health investigators were successful in persuading numerous Hollywood producers to include messages about "designated drivers" in popular television shows (Winsten, 1994). Following this effort, public opinion surveys showed increased public awareness and acceptance of the concept. In effect, the media were useful in this strategy in establishing a new health behavior norm.

Public service advertising is a common use of the media by many public health campaigns. To fulfill their public service obligations, most television and other broadcast stations devote free time to airing brief public service announcements (PSAs), usually 60 seconds or less. PSAs can play important roles as components of multistrategy, community-based public health campaigns. On one level, PSAs can help to define a public health problem as an important issue worthy of attention by community groups and institutions. This is the use of PSAs in building the community agenda of important public issues (Carter, Stamm, & Heintz-Knowles, 1992; Hilgartner & Bosk, 1988; McKinlay, 1993; Siska, Jason, Murdoch, Yang, & Donovan, 1992; Weiss & Tschirhart, 1994). On another level, PSAs can provide individuals with brief messages that not only raise issue salience but describe and urge specific actions to ameliorate the problem and to reduce personal risk. This is the use of PSAs to promote individual cognitive and behavioral impact (Bandura, 1994; Burdus, 1990). Community-based public health campaigns do not rely solely on PSAs but seek to integrate them into a "total communication" strategy.

The Future

The media system in the United States and worldwide is in a dramatic state of change and growth that offers both advantages and disadvantages to its use in public health campaigns. For example, in the United States since the early 1980s, we have witnessed an explosion in the availability of multichannel television through cable, satellite, and digital broadcasting. Videocassette technology has grown with equal vigor. At this writing, even telephone and electric companies are contemplating entering the market with media entertainment, advertising, and news services. The preponderance of the personal computer is rapidly blurring the lines between traditional print and electronic media. Computer-based environments such as the World Wide Web offer phenomenal amounts of information and entertainment on demand in multimedia formats that defy the traditional separation of print and electronic media. Some commentators have even called this change a movement from "mass" to "interactive" media (Chamberlain, 1996).

Public health has barely begun to use this new capacity in community-based campaigns, and we can only guess where its evolution may lead, but we may speculate that its potential is exciting for health promotion. True interactive media may offer the potential for greater end-user control and customization of content on demand. It may also offer real-time interaction with health educators and public health advocates in "virtual" communities. Even the World Wide Web, as currently configured, may offer training to communities in the various strategies of health promotion to help address particular public health problems. New media may thus be useful in disseminating intervention strategies and experience from community-based research projects to a much broader, nonprofessional audience.

Although these speculations offer much to think about by way of new media uses in health promotion, there will continue to be some older, more persistent concerns that will need to be addressed. Key among these are continuing SES-based gaps in media access, exposure, use, and impact. Evidence strongly suggests that SES differentials result not only in "knowledge gaps" but in serious differences in health outcomes and quality of life (Winkleby, 1994, 1997; Winkleby, Fortmann, & Barrett, 1990; Winkleby, Fortmann, & Rockhill, 1992; Winkleby, Jatulis, Frank, & Fortmann, 1992). The media, of course, are only a contributing factor to these inequalities, but unless serious attention is devoted to overcoming the communication barriers based in social structural differences, we will not be able to claim success in community-based health promotion except with the most advantaged groups.

CHAPTER 6

Evaluating Community Health Promotion Programs

Basic Questions and Approaches

PHYLLIS L. PIRIE

Community programs, like other health and human service programs, are increasingly under pressure to evaluate their activities and to demonstrate the value of what they do. Stakeholders of all types—from funders and boards of directors through program staff and professional colleagues—have adopted the language of evaluation and routinely ask for evaluation plans. Exactly what they are asking for varies from one setting to another, however, and is often not clearly defined. This chapter has two purposes: first, to provide a brief overview of types of evaluation questions that are typically asked and the types of stakeholders who are likely to ask each question and, second, to highlight some issues in the evaluation of community programs that are different from the evaluation of other types of health promotion programs.

Types of Evaluation Questions

Those responsible for community health promotion programs encounter a variety of pressures to evaluate their programs. Requests for evaluation are most often made by funding agencies, boards of directors, program staff who want information to guide their activities, and professional peers who would like to replicate a program. These groups all have slightly different questions and evaluation needs, and it is useful to sort out the types of questions they are asking before deciding how to proceed with an evaluation.

The pressures to evaluate generally fall into one of three basic types. Evaluation for accountability is the type most often requested by funding agencies and boards of directors, who want to know generally whether the expenditure of funds for the program is worthwhile and who will ultimately decide whether to continue funding or supporting the program. Evaluation for program improvement is most often the concern of management and staff, who are concerned about where to concentrate their efforts and about the success of their various activities and who want to decide whether to make changes in the program. Evaluation for generalizability is desired by academic and professional peers, who want to know whether programs of this type are generally useful and whether this specific program should be copied or disseminated. Questions about generalizability may also be important to policy makers in deciding whether to publicize, advocate, or market the program.

Despite the emphasis on asking evaluation questions that are relevant to decision making, everyone concerned with evaluation in a professional capacity quickly comes to realize that evaluation results are only one of many inputs into programmatic decisions. Decisions are affected as much or more by budgetary considerations, political considerations (for example, pressures from community members, clients, and other organizations), staffing considerations, and larger organizational priorities. Nevertheless, evaluation results can be useful, either by directly influencing decisions about specific programs or by influencing general thinking about types of programs. The goal should always be to plan to produce a useful evaluation, even though that goal won't always be reached.

EVALUATIONS AND EVALUATION QUESTIONS
WHILE PROGRAMS ARE BEING PLANNED

Even while programs are being planned, those with evaluation skills may be called on to contribute information that can be useful in determining the shape and direction of the program. These types of data collection activities are generally titled *needs assessment, community assessment*, and *formative studies* (although the term *formative evaluation* is sometimes used in a broader sense, to refer to *process evaluation*). Needs assessments and community assessments are most often requested by funding agencies and other policy-level decision makers, who want to justify the proposed expenditures. Program management and staff may ask for formative studies, which help them produce quality materials.

Needs assessments generally ask questions about the overall need or rationale for the program. How big is the problem that the program will address? What are the characteristics of those affected? What is the problem's cost to the community, either in terms of health care costs, social services, or human suffering? Are there other programs already addressing this problem, and are there gaps in what they are doing? Are there gaps between what people in the community know, think, or understand, and what they need to know, think, or understand to maximize health? Community assessments are similar but focus on a more broadly defined array of needs within a specified community, asking questions such as, What are the problems or unmet needs in this community? What resources already exist to address these needs? What other resources are needed? Data for both needs assessments and community assessments generally come from community surveys, compiled health or social statistics, and rosters of community services.

Formative evaluation, in the sense used by media researchers (Cambre, 1981), is used to judge the appropriateness of educational or promotional materials and is particularly useful if it is carried out while the materials are being designed. Issues for formative evaluation include accuracy of content, appropriateness of language and/or reading level, attractiveness of models, interpretability of symbols, and general appeal of the material.

Strategies for formative evaluation of health promotion media have included expert panels, focus groups, and in-depth interviews. Expert panels may be asked to comment on the accuracy of the information contained in the materials. Individuals drawn from the target audience for the materials may be asked to examine the materials; they are then tested to indicate their comprehension of the information. Focus groups may be asked to describe more qualitative responses such as their interpretation of drawings and symbols. All of these procedures are carried out while the materials are in production, so that changes can be made before the product is finalized.

EVALUATIONS AND EVALUATION QUESTIONS
WHILE PROGRAMS ARE UNDER WAY

Once the program is under way, the compelling questions to be addressed are questions concerning whether the program is operating as expected. This type of evaluation is generally labeled program or process evaluation. Process evaluation is most often the type desired by program management and staff, whose major concerns are with operating programs efficiently, meeting programmatic goals, and satisfying clients. Professional peers who wish to replicate a program may also be concerned with some aspects of process evaluation.

Perhaps the most basic process evaluation question is, Is the program being implemented as planned? Getting an answer to this question is usually tedious and time consuming. The question implies that there is a clearly specified plan of what exactly should occur. Although such a plan may exist, it is often not written down in any one location, so that an important first step for the evaluator is to document the program. Documenting the program not only can help improve the operation of the program but also can help interpret the outcome evaluation and serve as a template for replicating the program. If a program achieved good outcomes, those wishing to replicate the program will need a clear description of exactly what was done. If the program did not achieve good outcomes, it is important to be able to differentiate inadequate theory from inadequate implementation.

Monitoring program implementation often includes review of existing program records but may involve the creation of new types of records or systems of recording, or it may involve interviews with participants or direct observations.

A related question to be addressed by process evaluation is, Is the program reaching its target audience? This is a key question for community-based health promotion programs, which frequently must market themselves in a public arena rather than finding a ready-made audience in a school or hospital setting. Getting a usable answer to this question implies that there are prior expectations regarding the target audience. As with questions about program operations, often the first task of the evaluator is to understand and document the expectations program managers have about the size and characteristics of their target audience.

Counting and characterizing the audience can be accomplished easily in a program that has a formal sign-up procedure but is much more difficult in the case of broad-based community activities such as the introduction of new smoking policies or programs that place nutrition information in grocery stores and restaurants. Some information about who is aware of these activities and their demographic characteristics can be obtained by on-the-spot interviews, for example with patrons of the grocery stores and restaurants involved in the programs. More precise information about the number and percent of individuals aware of such programs can be gained only from population-based surveys, which are an expensive data collection strategy. Audience characteristics for media programs can sometimes be learned from commercial ratings services.

A slightly different but related question is, Who is the program failing to reach, and why? Sometimes a very useful appraisal of the program's ability to reach its audience can be obtained by assessing people who might have been expected to take part but did not. Were they unaware of the program? Were they aware but found the program unappealing? Did they fail to perceive their own need to take part? Answers to these questions can have direct implications for improving the program.

Obtaining data about nonparticipants can be difficult in many circumstances. One major problem is to identify a population of nonparticipants. Program dropouts are one part of this population and can often be identified and surveyed, but they do not represent those who were unaware of the program or found it too unappealing even to sign up.

A final question that is often an important focus of process evaluation is, Are the program's participants satisfied with their experience? Interest in this question is often driven partly by an organization's need to satisfy the "consumers" of a program, in the hope that they will return for other programs or recommend the organization's programs to others. Another rationale for asking the question is the premise (never clearly demonstrated for health promotion programs) that satisfied participants will have more positive outcomes. For these reasons, participant ratings of satisfaction are one of the most commonly performed types of evaluation. Unfortunately, the results are less useful than one might think. A major problem underlying these evaluations is a positive ratings bias (Stipak, 1980): Program participants generally rate their experience as satisfactory, particularly for programs that are voluntary in nature. Various explanations have been advanced to explain this phenomenon: cognitive consistency (that participants are reluctant to downgrade a program on which they have spent time, money, or energy), self-selection into programs (that participants select only those programs that appear on the surface to meet their particular needs), or a general response style of not wishing to appear critical or ungrateful. This positive bias does not mean that participant ratings are useless but that such evaluations should be carefully designed and the results carefully interpreted.

A key issue in interpreting all process evaluation results is having an established standard that can be used for comparison. For example, program participation may be compared to an established participation goal or to participation rates in similar programs; implementation can most usefully be assessed against a fixed standard plan for implementation. Similarly, interpretation of satisfaction data is facilitated if a standard for comparison is clearly established. Do the program planners wish to achieve a set level of satisfaction on a standard set of questions, or achieve satisfaction that is comparable to or better than that achieved in similar programs? Or perhaps the comparisons are between different aspects of the program, so that the aspect given the lowest satisfaction rating is examined for improvement even if the absolute level of satisfaction is relatively high.

This list of potential questions that could be addressed in a process evaluation is lengthy, and obviously no single program will be evaluated on all of these questions. The process of determining which of these questions needs to be answered to improve a particular program will depend on the specific program and on concerns voiced by the program staff and relevant stakeholders.

Process evaluations should always involve a feedback loop, so that the information gained can quickly be used to improve the program. This is particularly critical for community-based programs, which are too expensive and too complex to be allowed to operate without the benefit of feedback and the opportunity to be "fine-tuned." Data need to be accumulated and examined in a timely fashion and reported rapidly to program managers, so adjustments can be made in program operations.

QUESTIONS ABOUT PROGRAM OUTCOMES

Finally, the evaluator may be asked to address questions regarding the program's outcomes: Is the program having the effect it is designed to have? Is any good resulting from this program? Outcome questions are often the first questions posed to the evaluator, but they should be the last ones to be answered. In general, outcome studies should not be conducted unless process evaluation has clearly demonstrated that the program is functioning as planned; otherwise, one risks making what Basch, Sliepcevich, Gold, Duncan, and Kolbe (1985) have labeled a "Type 3 error," that is, evaluating a program that doesn't exist. Outcome studies generally are most called for when the core question is one of accountability; outcome studies usually provide relatively little information that can be used for fine-tuning and improving programs. Professional colleagues interested in replicating a program are another likely audience for outcome evaluation.

Deciding what is meant by program "outcomes" or "effects" is often more difficult than it would first appear. A single program is likely to have multiple effects. For example, a smoking cessation program for pregnant women may have effects ranging from changes in maternal knowledge through maternal smoking, infant birthweight, and even infant morbidity. Thus, the "outcome" of the program could be evaluated with regard to any of these effects. The choice of which outcome to study is determined by several factors: the strength of the scientific evidence linking the various effects (e.g., as the relationship of infant birthweight to morbidity is well established, evaluating birthweight alone may be considered sufficient), the feasibility and cost of obtaining the measurement (maternal outcomes may be more feasible to obtain than infant outcomes in some settings), and the statistical power to detect effects at various levels (due to considerations of measurement variability, it may be statistically easier to detect differences in infant birthweight than differences in subsequent morbidity). The choice of which endpoint to measure is also dependent upon the needs of the audience for the evaluation: For example, will the program's directors be satisfied if smoking cessation is demonstrated, or do they need to see evidence pertaining to infant birthweight before they are convinced of the utility of the program? Often, more than one effect is measured (e.g., both smoking cessation and birthweight are monitored). In many cases, however, tensions exist regarding the choice of effects to be evaluated; frequently, program directors and boards request information on outcomes that are more distal than the evaluator thinks is practical or realistic. These cases require careful negotiation and marshaling of scientific and statistical evidence to develop a sound decision on the choice of endpoints.

Identifying the important outcomes or effects is, of course, only the first step in thinking about an outcome evaluation. Just as process evaluation data are best interpreted by making use of the logic of comparisons, outcome evaluations are also based on the use of comparisons. We are always asking the question, What would have been the outcome in this community if the program had not been in place? Strictly speaking, that question is unanswerable; research designs are devices that attempt to provide an answer by providing a way to estimate what the outcome would have been without the program. That outcome is sometimes approximated by examining the outcome measure in the community before the program took place, or by looking at the outcome measure in similar communities without the program. The first design is sometimes called a "pre-post," or before and after, comparison and is particularly weak in the case of a community program because so much is happening to the community other than the community program itself. In other words, it is difficult to be sure that the change that is observed is due to the program. The second design—comparison to similar communities without the program—can be much stronger, although steps must be taken to be certain that the communities are in fact comparable in every respect except for the introduction of the community program.

Issues Specific to the Evaluation of Community Programs

Much of the previous discussion is applicable to the evaluation of any large health promotion program. The evaluation of community programs generally follows the same underlying logic, but there are several unique features of community programs that raise specific issues for evaluation.

Because community programs are typically complex and involve many staff and a variety of activities, monitoring program implementation is particularly important. Computer-based record-keeping systems have been developed to allow staff and management to track their activities and to assure that those activities are consistent with program objectives (COMMIT Research Group, 1991; McGraw et al., 1988).

A defining characteristic of community programs is that they are interested in changing health-related behaviors and outcomes in entire communities, not just in an enrolled sample. A crucial issue for the success of the program is program penetration or exposure; that is, the proportion of community members who are aware of the message or take part in the activities of the program. Even very powerful health promotion programs will fail to have an impact on a community if they are not sufficiently well attended. Thus, the measurement of program exposure as an aspect of process evaluation requires considerable attention. Community health promotion programs have followed the lead of media researchers in conceptualizing the evaluation of program exposure as consisting of two parts: delivered dose (what messages or events the program delivered and to whom) and received dose (how many people received the messages or took part in the events). Specific methodologies have been developed for measuring exposure in community-based programs (Finnegan, Murray, Kurth, & McCarthy, 1989; McGraw et al., 1988).

Another issue specific to the evaluation of community programs is that short-term impacts of the program sometimes need to be measured at a level other than the individual. For example, the program might hypothesize that it brings about change by changing the organizations in the community, which in turn will affect community residents. Thus evaluation measures need to assess the affected community organizations, which might include schools, worksites, churches, and places of business. Methodology for sampling and measuring these changes is less well developed than methodology for sampling and measuring individual changes, and much remains to be done to maximize the potential of these measures (Cheadle et al., 1990; Weisbrod, Pirie, & Bracht, 1992).

Outcome evaluation of community programs also has its own array of difficulties. In keeping with the community program's emphasis on whole communities, outcomes are generally assessed on samples of community members drawn at random or in another way selected to be representative of the community as a whole rather than being assessed on active program participants. This can lead to difficulties, both in obtaining cooperation for the assessment procedure and in explaining the logic of the assessment to staff.

A particularly difficult consideration for evaluation of community programs is the design of the outcome evaluation. As discussed above, the strongest design for outcome evaluation of community programs is a design that compares the outcome in the program community to the outcome in a similar community that did not receive the program (called the control or comparison community). Recent work on designs for evaluating community programs has led to increasing awareness of the need to incorporate multiple community pairs into valid designs for outcome evaluations (Murray, 1995). Although earlier community programs were often based on comparisons of a single program community to a single comparison community, or at most a comparison of two or three pairs of program and comparison communities, recent thinking about the statistical aspects of this design has led to the awareness that a valid comparison of communities will involve a larger number of pairs—often on the order of 10 or more pairs. The COMMIT trial of smoking cessation, for example, used 11 matched pairs of communities in different parts of the country (COMMIT Research Group, 1991). Thus the outcome evaluation of community programs has become an expensive proposition that needs significant foresight and planning so that it may be implemented in a meaningful way.

The statistical issues involved in calculating the number of communities needed can be daunting, but it is easy to understand on an intuitive level why multiple communities are needed to clearly interpret the effects caused by a community program. Each individual community is essentially one example of program implementation; if a mass media campaign goes awry, for example, it goes awry for the entire community; if it is implemented spectacularly well, it is implemented spectacularly well for the entire community. Therefore, to understand the typical impact of the planned mass media campaign, one needs to have multiple examples of its implementation in multiple communities.

Another issue specific to the outcome evaluation of community programs is knowing what is going on in the comparison communities. Unlike a typical "research trial," in which one can be confident that the comparison group is not receiving the intervention, in community trials we are often uncertain of what exactly is happening in the comparison communities. Recent research has tended to show an upsurge in health promotion programs of all types in many communities. In many cases, when researchers have attempted to analyze the "dose" of health promotion programming in the intervention communities as compared to the control communities, it has been remarkably difficult to demonstrate a difference (Luepker et al., 1994; Weisbrod et al., 1992). Not being aware of this difficulty means that the evaluator risks naively comparing outcomes across communities that have received essentially similar doses of programming. An ongoing series of community assessments, applied to the comparison communities as well as the intervention communities, can be used to monitor the "dose" of health promotion programming in both sets of communities. These are most useful for monitoring purposes if they are quantified so that comparisons can be made (Weisbrod et al., 1992).

Carrying Out Evaluation Studies

Carrying out evaluation studies requires strong technical skills in research and evaluation methods, and certainly outcome studies should not be attempted without involving staff or consultants who have considerable expertise in measurement methods as well as statistical design and analysis techniques. The issues are the same issues encountered in social research of all types: For example, What is the design? (Are there comparison groups? How are they chosen? When are measurements taken?); How are data to be collected? (questionnaire, interview, observation); What is the quality of the data collection instrument? (reliability, validity); and How are the data to be processed and analyzed? A large body of knowledge has accumulated regarding the best way to make such choices: The principles are taught in numerous courses, articles, and textbooks (e.g., Cook & Campbell, 1979; Windsor, Baranowski, Clark, & Cutter, 1994), and if expertise to make these choices and carry out the evaluation is not available within the program, it can usually be obtained by hiring outside consultants. University departments of social and behavioral science are often good sources of advice and consultation on such issues, although there are also many private evaluation consulting firms who have considerable expertise in these issues.

Although there are many technical considerations in planning and carrying out process evaluation and planning studies, the design and statistical analyses are somewhat less complex and are often carried out by individuals with less experience, although the consultation of an experienced evaluator will almost always prove beneficial. The most useful information will always result when the purpose of the information and the specific questions to be answered are well formulated in advance, and achieving this clarity of purpose is often the joint mission of program staff and the evaluator.

Summary

Although the prospect of evaluating something as large and complex as a community-based health promotion program may seem daunting, the key to a good evaluation is clear thinking about the purpose of the evaluation. The first step in planning the evaluation is asking who needs the information and for what purpose, and how will the information be used? With the answers to these questions firmly in mind, the more technical aspects of planning and carrying out the evaluation can be conducted either in-house or by an external evaluator, depending on the availability of appropriate expertise. Whoever is charged with conducting the evaluation should be aware of issues specific to the evaluation of community programs, which differ somewhat from the evaluation of other health promotion programs.

PART II

Cross-National Experiences: Issues in Developing and Sustaining Community Health Programs

CHAPTER 7

Durability of Community Intervention Programs

Definitions, Empirical Studies, and Strategic Planning

BETI THOMPSON

CAROL WINNER

Grant-funded community research projects are primarily interested in answering one question: Does the intervention have an effect? The efficacy or effectiveness of an intervention may, however, lead to related questions: Will the effect last? Will long-term behavior change be seen? Will the intervention program endure? The last question is very important, as funding agencies increasingly view their resources as "seed money" to support intervention while a community builds an infrastructure to continue such activities after the external funding ends (Altman, 1995; ASSIST Working Group on Durability, 1996; COMMIT Research Group, 1991; Tarlov et al., 1987). Similarly, there is a belief that communities that have been involved in addressing a public health problem will have both the wish and enhanced capacity to continue activities at some level (Altman, 1995; Altman et al., 1991; Florin & Wandersman, 1990; Green, 1986; Jackson et al., 1994; Kelly, 1979; Tarlov et al., 1987; Rifkin, 1986; Wallack & Wallerstein, 1986).

For some years, numerous community research studies have formed partnerships with community members (Abramson, Gofin, Hopp, Donchin, & Habib, 1981; COMMIT Research Group, 1991; Dwyer, Pierce, Hannam, & Burke, 1986; Egger et al., 1983; Elder et al., 1986; Farquhar, Fortmann, et al., 1985; Farquhar, Maccoby, et al., 1977; Gutzwiller, Nater, & Martin, 1985; Maccoby, Farquhar, Wood, & Alexander, 1977; McAlister, Puska, Salonen, Toumilehto, & Koskela, 1982; Stunkard, Felix, Yopp, & Cohen, 1985). Based on community organization strategies and the principle of participation (see Chapters 2 and 4), the research studies have involved community partners at various levels ranging from a group that supports the research agenda but has little decision-making power to almost autonomous boards or coalitions that are involved in all aspects of decision making. The majority of research projects, however, try to strike a balance between community and research needs (Mittelmark, 1990). Community partners who perceive some good coming out of the project often wish to have the means for project durability (Altman et al., 1991; Bossert, 1990; Bracht, Finnegan, et al., 1994; Lefebvre, 1990a; Lichtenstein, Thompson, Nettekoven, & Corbett, 1996; Rifkin, 1986; Wandersman & Florin, 1990). Unfortunately, many research organizations have simply removed themselves after the research phase of the project has ended, leaving the community partners without resources, capabilities, or other avenues to address the original problem. Such an action on the part of researchers is considered inconsistent with the principles of community ownership and partnership (Green, 1986; Green & McAlister, 1984; Thompson & Kinne, 1990; Thompson, Lichtenstein, Wallack, & Pehacek, 1990-1991; Wallack & Wallerstein, 1986).

There are a number of reasons that may explain why little effort is made to encourage ongoing intervention at the conclusion of a research project. The first is that the answer to the question of project effectiveness may not be known by the end of the intervention phase. In trials where final data are gathered postintervention, the data collection, cleaning, and analysis phases may be lengthy and significant time may elapse before the trialwide result is known (Carleton et al., 1995; COMMIT Research Group, 1995). Researchers are often reluctant to continue activities that may not be efficacious.

Another potential explanation is that researchers do not build in either time or activities to promote durability. The realities of dealing with community projects that are often complex and time-consuming may make it difficult to maintain pace with the research activities, providing little time or energy for planning for the future. Only recently have some trials built in transition time and resources to plan for activities beyond the research years (ASSIST Working Group on Durability, 1996). Finally, it may be that too little is known about the process or the skills needed for planning for durability (Florin & Wandersman, 1990; Wandersman & Florin, 1990).

Community members often have a wish to continue intervention activities even when the results of a trial are ambiguous or unknown. In the Community Intervention Trial for Smoking Cessation (COMMIT), for example, a durability assessment of the intervention communities only (described below) was conducted before trial results were known, and yet community members were very enthusiastic about continuing tobacco control activities (Lichtenstein et al., 1996). Similarly, the Bloomington Heart Health Board continues with some modifications 17 years after its initiation into the Minnesota Heart Health Program, despite the mixed results of the overall project (see Chapter 1 and Bracht, Finnegan, et al., 1994). Why is there an emphasis on continuing such activities? One answer might lie in the creeping pace at which human behavior change takes place. Behavioral change at the population level may begin with a small change that increases over time (Beresford et al., 1997; Henderson, Thompson, & Kristal, 1995; Puska, Salonen, Nissinen, & Tuomilehto, 1983; Puska, Tuomilehto, et al., 1979). Long-lasting and widespread behavior changes require modifications in social norms to incorporate the behavior into society. Behavior change that occurs at the community level may increase as time goes on because change that affects the prevalence of a certain behavior in a community is also likely to affect community norms, which will lead to ever greater change in the community. This often requires more time than research projects allow. The North Karelia project, for example, did not see changes in smoking behavior until 10 years after the project was initiated (Puska, Salonen, et al., 1983; Puska, Tuomilehto, et al., 1979). COMMIT did not begin to see results in smoking cessation until 3 years after the communities were randomized (COMMIT Research Group, 1995).

Some community intervention studies have demonstrated positive effects (Abramson et al., 1981; COMMIT Research Group, 1995; Fortmann, Taylor, Flora, & Jatulis, 1993; Gutzwiller, Nater, & Martin, 1985; Kornitzer, Dramaix, Kittel, & DeBacker, 1980; Lando et al., 1995; Macaskill, Pierce, Simpson, & Lyle, 1992; Puska et al., 1983; Steenkamp, Jooste, Jordaan, Swanepoel, & Rossouw, 1991). When such effects are seen, it is crucial to continue intervention activities in some form to perpetuate change. Some researchers have summarized it well when they note that research findings must be *applied* to have a public health effect (Altman et al., 1991). Application often takes the form of assisting communities in intervention maintenance. Although described in various ways, perhaps the best descriptor of this process is "capacity-building" of the community to continue activities by itself, which will sustain social environmental and behavioral changes once the researchers have left (Green, 1986; Jackson et al., 1994). In this chapter, we examine definitions of durability, studies of durability, and ideas for strategic planning for durability.

Definitions of Durability

There is considerable divergence of opinion as to the appropriate word to be used to describe some maintenance of project activities after the initial researchers have left the community. The different words may have slightly different nuances of meaning; however, they have many similarities.

INSTITUTIONALIZATION

Institutionalization is probably the most commonly used word to express maintenance of intervention activities (Buller & McEvoy, 1989; Goodman, McLeroy, Steckler, & Hoyle, 1993; Goodman & Steckler, 1987; Goodman & Steckler, 1988-1989; Goodman & Steckler, 1990; Steckler & Goodman, 1989). It refers to the process whereby a program continues on its own, usually within an existing organization. The majority of research done on institutionalization focuses on a program becoming an accepted part of an organization's mission with resources allocated for the program (Goodman & Steckler, 1987; Terborg, 1988). In a review of 10 case studies of nonprofit organizations, Steckler and Goodman (1989) identified six factors related to the successful institutionalization of an intervention program. These were (a) programs that found a "champion" to promote the program, (b) programs that were placed in organizations with strong subsystems, (c) programs that had a good fit with the organizational mission, (d) programs where funds went directly to an organization and not through an intermediary, (e) programs with funding for a sufficiently long time, and (f) funding of existing programs rather than the development of new programs. Institutionalization may be threatened when these factors are not present. In one case study, a nationally recognized substance abuse project was not institutionalized because funds ended and the program was seen as being "dumped" into an organization with scarce resources (Goodman & Steckler, 1988-1989).

Although not identical to institutionalization as defined above, a similar approach to the survival of programs in neighborhoods has been described by Wandersman and Florin (1990). In their work with neighborhoods and neighborhood block programs, they found that the most likely to survive are those that develop organizational structures, have a task focus, and have a process for filling roles. This approach builds largely on citizen participation and empowerment and views success in those areas as leading to long-term community development (Florin & Wandersman, 1990). Others have noted the difficulty of attaining community development, especially in the United States, where communities tend to be heterogeneous and have to raise their own revenues for health promotion activities (Heller, 1990). Recognition of this and other factors has led Wandersman and Florin (1990) to encourage that community development activities be maintained in a single organization that is strikingly similar to the definition of institutionalization.

INCORPORATION

Institutionalization is increasingly used to mean the continuation of program activities within an existing organization. This may be problematic for community studies where many groups and organizations may be involved in intervention activities (Mittelmark, Hunt, Heath, & Schmid, 1993). In the Minnesota Heart Health Program (MHHP), the term *incorporation* was used to overcome the potential limitations of institutionalization. Incorporation was defined as the "maintenance of specific intervention program types over time, after external funding resources (Bracht, Finnegan, et al., 1994). Program activities were considered incorporated if (a) a local provider continued the original program, (b) a local provider continued the program in a modified way, or (c) a local provider continued the program but offered it only occasionally (Bracht, Finnegan, et al., 1994). The distinction between institutionalization and incorporation at the community level appears to be that programs may be continued by many providers and that programs may undergo modification and still be considered to have some fidelity to the original intervention activities.

SUSTAINABILITY

A term that is more commonly used outside of the United States is *sustainability*, which generally refers to the ability of a program to continue delivering activities and benefits after external assistance ends (Altman, 1995; Bossert, 1990; LaFond, 1995, Lefebvre, 1992). This definition is primarily used in the field of community development and may refer to the ability of developing nations to fold intervention programs into existing government agencies and agendas. Bossert (1990), for example, examined the sustainability of health projects in Africa and Central America and concluded that sustainability was closely related to the economic, political, and institutional contexts of developing countries, with more stable countries more likely to sustain intervention programs. (Chapters that follow in Part II of this book provide examples and discussions of experiences with sustainability.)

In another set of five case studies (Nepal, Uganda, Pakistan, Ghana, and Vietnam), economic conditions, political climate, the aid system, and the market were related to sustainability (LaFond,

1995). In that review, a stable economic environment was more likely to sustain programs; furthermore, the higher the earnings of a country, the higher the public health care expenditures. Local political climates were seen to be as important as the national climate because breakdowns in delivery of a program often occurred at the local level. The aid system must respond to both donors and recipients, with many donors requiring strict conditions relating to the distribution of aid. (A good example of this can be found in examples of aid from the United States in which the U.S. Congress demands that the results of the aid be clearly visible to the American public. Similarly, the U.S. Congress generally limits aid to a short time period—3 to 5 years—making it difficult to plan long-term change strategies.) Programs that pay attention to marketing their services appear to do better than those that simply assume people will take advantage of offered services. This is especially important in environments where traditional cultural practices may clash with Western medicine (LaFond, 1995).

Some researchers in the United States also have used *sustainability* as a term of ongoing maintenance. Altman (1995) captures many dimensions by defining sustainability as the "infrastructure" that remains after research activities are concluded. In his view, this includes (a) the maintenance of interventions, (b) the modification of organizations as a result of being part of a research study, and (c) the diffusion of skills gained by individuals in other aspects of their lives. It is also important to increase a community's capacity to deal with issues, as this ability is a good measure of sustainability (Altman, 1995).

CAPACITY BUILDING

A similar theme is found in the term *capacity building*. Going back to the roots of community organization and empowerment, proponents of this term argue that once the community has the capacity to address its own problems or issues, the community will decide what is important to maintain. The Stanford Five-City Study that intervened in cardiovascular disease risk factors concluded that such capacity building could be defined as the degree to which community members or organizations had the knowledge, resources, and skills to carry out programs (Jackson et al., 1994).

DURABILITY

A relatively new term in the literature is *durability*. The term has developed in recognition that after a research study ends, what remains in the community may take many forms (ASSIST Working Group on Durability, 1996; Bracht, Thompson, & Winner, 1996; Lichtenstein et al., 1996). It may be that some activities or policies are incorporated into organizations; others may become integral to some institutions; still others may become part of the normative climate of the community. Although more amorphous than some of the other terms defined in this section, *durability* will be used in this chapter because of its flexibility. *Durability* may be defined as the maintenance of some degree of activity in an area around which a community was mobilized to take action as a result of a research project. Thus, durability may fall upon a continuum where it is as specific as continuing one activity in an organization or as broad as a political change in a law, ordinance, or policy that changes the social environment (e.g., restrictions on tobacco access or use; requirements that children receive vaccinations to attend school). Durability does not require that specific intervention activities be continued or that specific organizations take on intervention activities. It does require that some sort of infrastructure or capacity be present to address the initial area of concern (unless, of course, the entire problem has disappeared, as has been the case with a few infectious diseases such as smallpox). A critical aspect of this definition is that durability can take many forms and assessment of durability should take that into account.

Past Studies and Examples of Durability

NATIONAL

Few studies have examined the long-term continuation of research project effects (see Chapter 1). Even fewer have examined the maintenance of project activities, and those focus on the intervention communities alone without evaluating what was happening in the control communities. The Minnesota Heart Health Project, for example, reported that 60% of intervention activities were incorporated in the three intervention communities 3 years after the educational intervention ended (Bracht, Finnegan, et al., 1994). During the late 1980s and early 1990s, however, there was much emphasis on health; in fact, the Minnesota investigators pointed to a strong secular trend as the reason for a large reduction of risk factors in the comparison communities. The comparison communities were not assessed in terms of similar programs and activities, so it is not clear that the intervention activities maintained in the three intervention communities were different from the control communities. The Stanford Five-City Project focused on capacity building and reported that a number of individuals in one community attended training sessions and achieved some success in generating grants and becoming a model test site (Jackson et al., 1994). Again, it is not clear how the nonintervention comparison communities fared. A report of tobacco control activities in the 11 intervention communities only of the Community Intervention Trial for Smoking Cessation (COMMIT) trial 12 months after the end of intervention activities indicated that respondents perceived substantial durability of COMMIT activities (Lichtenstein et al., 1996). However, a recent study that examined the tobacco control activities of the 11 COMMIT intervention and the 11 control communities 2 years after intervention ended indicated very little difference in tobacco control activities between intervention and control communities; both types of communities had considerable tobacco control activities (Thompson, Lichtenstein, Corbett, Nettekoven, & Feng, 1998). Interestingly, despite an overall lack of difference, respondents in the intervention communities thought a considerable amount of activity remained from the COMMIT trial.

The United States has produced community research studies that tend to be time limited and without a focus on durability. For many community projects, durability has tended to be an "add-on" while the intervention is ending. As previously mentioned, research projects that include U.S. aid to developing countries suffer from the same time limitations, making it difficult to establish a durable project.

INTERNATIONAL

Some countries outside of the United States have fared better in achieving durability. Primarily this may be attributed to different approaches to health taken by other countries. In Finland, for example, there was national concern over the high rates of cardiovascular disease in North Karelia, a county in eastern Finland (Puska, Salonen, et al., 1983). The North Karelia study that was developed and tested as a result of the concern was long term (10 years), and the sponsors expected to apply the program to other settings if the results were favorable (Puska, Salonen, et al., 1983). Indeed, a major goal of the project was to find ways for communities to control the cardiovascular epidemic.

Other countries may build research components into ongoing programs that address health. In Sweden, the national Health and Medical Services Act requires county councils to promote the health of its constituents. In response, Stockholm County formed the Stockholm Cancer Prevention Program (SCPP). The project, which began in 1987, is scheduled to continue at least to the year 2000. The project directors have taken advantage of the Scandinavian emphasis on health to build a comprehensive cancer prevention intervention and research program into the national agenda (Holm, 1991).

Some European countries in particular have established systems for easily intervening in some new area, thereby having some of the infrastructure characteristics considered important for durability. Norway, for example, used the well-established national tuberculosis prevention program to intervene in cardiovascular risk factors (Bjarveit, 1986). The durability of the program is the structure left in place for other intervention areas in the future (see following chapters for examples).

Health programs in the developing world are less likely to evolve into strong durable programs. Some of the reasons have already been discussed (e.g., contextual factors, instability, short-term assistance). Another potential reason is that community members are rarely involved in health programs beyond being recipients of such programs (Rifkin, 1986). Even in instances where community members are trained to provide primary health care, only a small portion of the citizenry is involved in a health program, providing little infrastructure or capacity for ongoing activities (LaFond, 1995; Rifkin, 1986).

Before leaving the area of research on durability, it is worth mentioning that some public health advocates recommend the implementation and sustaining of preventive action without testing intervention programs at the community level (Atwood, Colditz, & Kawachi, 1997). Arguing that public health science often far precedes prevention, proponents of early widespread implementation note that only three components need to be present to produce prevention: knowledge, the political will to support change, and strategies to achieve change (Atwood et al., 1997). Indeed, community smoking prevention trials are taken to task for insisting on rigorous scientific research (i.e., randomized community trials) for allowing "scientific integrity [to] outstrip social relevance" (Atwood et al., 1997, p. 1604). The implications of such an approach on the definition and assessment of durability are great; presumably, community trials would not be necessary because the knowledge could be obtained from other types of trials. Despite such arguments, it is unlikely that the scientific community will support the implementation of interventions without a controlled test; similarly, it is unlikely that the sponsors in the United States will provide long-term support for untested programs. Thus, we may cautiously conclude that

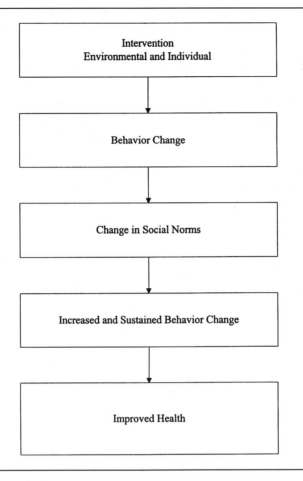

Figure 7.1. Objectives of Community Intervention Projects

programs that have the best chance to remain at some level are those that have been tested and have been shown to be effective.

Strategic Planning for Durability

MOTIVATION FOR CONTINUING ACTIVITIES

Why do people become involved in health promotion projects? We know there are huge human, financial, and public health burdens associated with unhealthy lifestyles and poor health. But knowledge of the problem does not predict participation in activities that are thought to lead to solutions. Something more is involved. That something is a basic belief that behavior change can be attained. Figure 7.1 illustrates a commonly held view of the pathway of intervention and human behavior change. As interventions are developed at both the societal and the individual level, behavior change occurs.

When enough behavior change occurs, those new behaviors become part of the social norms of our everyday life; that is, the rules people live by. As the behavior becomes more normative, more people incorporate the change as part of their lives and increased behavior change is seen. Just as important is the point that the behavior change becomes sustained over time, so more people are behaving in a healthy way. That, ultimately, leads to improved health in society. Many people become involved in social projects because of beliefs that something can be done to improve the public health in society.

Individuals who believe they can make a difference become involved in many different change agents, including coalitions, organizations, voluntary groups, government, and others. These groups are committed to activities that use strategies that will lead to widespread and long-lasting improved health.

By the time most research projects are ready to plan for durability, participants in the research project, whether they be community members, staff, or researchers, have already engaged in considerable planning just to make the research project operate. What makes planning for durability different? First, there is not a protocol or even guidelines to define what needs to be done after the research ends. Second, even the concept of durability is rather vague. What should last? All of the intervention activities? If not, how does one determine what the key intervention activities were? Third, the future is largely unknown, especially in terms of resources. After many years of being relatively secure in the knowledge that research funding would be forthcoming, community members now will have to grapple with ways to identify resources that can finance activities. And finally, some of the volunteers are tired and do not wish to continue the work. Strategic planning for durability will help to address these issues.

When people plan activities to change the social environment and/or behavior, they often make the mistake of thinking that the people to be changed are just like the people planning the activities (Heller, 1990). Even worse, they often assume that all the people targeted for change are the same. When projects are complicated and involve a number of individuals and groups in implementing the change activities, even the assumption that those groups are the same is usually untrue (Heller, 1990). This becomes very important in planning for the future.

A SYSTEM'S PERSPECTIVE OF STRATEGIC PLANNING

A basic assumption of strategic planning is that although individuals and groups are very different, they all exist in a "system" in which common goals and objectives can be developed. As shown in Figure 7.2, one might think of a system as a set of Ping-Pong balls held together by rubber bands. The Ping-Pong balls are quite solid and stable, but their linkages, the rubber bands, are flexible and likely to adjust to tugs and pulls on the Ping-Pong balls. Applying this image, all the balls together form the social environment within which we live. The connections between the balls are societal interrelationships, including consensus, compromise, and conflict. Some of the Ping-Pong balls are unlikely ever to adopt public health goals (e.g., the tobacco industry). Other

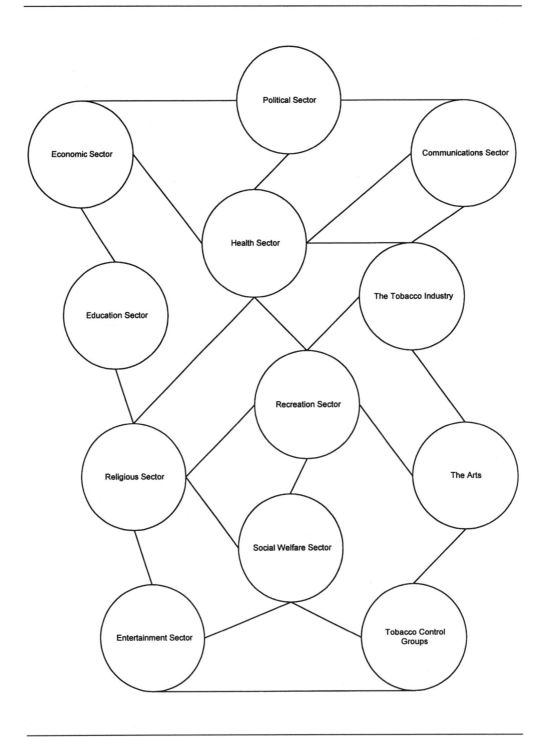

Figure 7.2. A Systems View of the Social Environment

Ping-Pong balls seem very peripherally related to public health goals (e.g., the arts sector). Other balls might have split allegiances (e.g., the political sector).

An important aspect of this way of looking at the social environment is that pressure on any part of the system will reverberate throughout the system. That actually is one of the aims of public health advocates: to change the system so the health of the public is promoted. We expect that this will have effects on the individuals within the system but also on entire sectors.

It is also obvious that the gain or loss of the support of any sector or part of a sector will have an influence on success. That is why it is strategically important to recruit other groups to participate in a change activity, especially those that, on the face of it, may not seem to have similar goals. For example, few individuals have thought of recruiting groups in the arts to assist in tobacco control. Noting however that the tobacco industry may sponsor art groups to legitimize their own image, tobacco control advocates have recognized the arts as an important sector to have on their side. Although the arts sector and the tobacco control sector have quite different overall goals and reasons for being involved in tobacco control activities, the result is a broader-based coalition for tobacco control. The systems approach is critical for understanding the importance of strategic planning.

Many kinds of planning techniques exist. Some organizations are locked into very rigid planning; for example, building contractors make very definite plans because their profit structure depends on the accuracy of the planning. When contractors encounter something unexpected, projects often go on hold while new plans and budgets are designed and renegotiated. Government agencies often have little opportunity to change their plans quickly because the planning is closely related to available finances. On the other hand, some organizations plan more loosely and take pride in being responsive to whatever situations might emerge. The Red Cross, with its quick response to emergencies, is an example. The very nature of the organization is to be prepared to take any action that may be needed.

Strategic planning is an approach that incorporates elements of all kinds of planning. It is "rigid" in the sense that members involved in the group or organization agree on the organization's overall goal. Going back to the Ping-Pong model, this means that members agree about the way they want the system to look. The goal may be general instead of very specific. Using the Red Cross example, the overall goal is to be responsive to emergencies, and the specifics of how to respond may vary by community, country, emergency, or other factors. A major difference between a strategic planning approach and other approaches is that strategic planning emphasizes flexibility. Thus, the way to get to a goal may follow different paths, depending on the social environment. Furthermore, the plan may change if the environment changes, if new barriers arise, if opportunities present themselves, or if new creative activities are found. In short, strategic planning responds to what is going on and is flexible enough to make changes over time (Hillebrand, 1994; Kinney & Gift, 1997; Weitekamp, Thorndyke, & Evarts, 1996).

Applying Strategic Planning Methods

The flexibility of strategic planning may sound somewhat confusing; fortunately, some basic questions help in planning. Responding to the questions will help identify potential problems that may arise over time. The questions revolve around the following concepts:

- Goal setting: Who participates in the activity of interest and why? Is the group diverse?
- Priorities: What are the most important outcomes to be reached?
- Barriers and facilitators: What factors will help or hinder one in reaching priorities and goals?
- Social environment: What social changes are looming on the horizon?
- Creativity: What new discoveries and applications may help?
- Flexibility: How can a "quick response" system be developed?

GOAL SETTING

There is no exhaustive list of who participates in any specific public health activity; each topic includes a number of "stakeholders" (interested parties) who participate for different reasons. Some people participate in some activities related to a project and not in others; other groups can always be depended on to participate. In planning for the future, it is necessary to identify who the main players were and who future players might be. It is essential to understand the basic goals that were held by all, even when people did not seem to agree on activities or priorities.

Equally important in planning for durability is the job of identifying new players. It is not realistic to expect volunteers to stay with a project forever. Recruiting new individuals and groups is a standard task for any volunteer organization; it is especially important to look outside of traditional areas and search out nontraditional players. There is no single answer to explain why an individual or group decides to participate in a project. Some do so because a project's emphasis is part of the organization's mandate. Others do so because they see some benefits that could be attained by their members. Others have a mission to provide community service. Others have no reason that they can state. Strategic planning requires identification of various current and potential participants.

PRIORITIES

Strategic planning emphasizes priority setting. Whatever the overall goal is, the priorities are seen and defined as the required objectives or steps needed to attain the goal. During the research portion of a project, the priorities are often set by the research. When planning for durability, it is wise to revisit the priorities using the information obtained from the research. Activities that were extremely labor- or resource-intensive may be less desirable than activities that are more efficient. Good strategic planning, however, also considers the impact of various activities. An efficient activity that has little impact on behavior or normative change must be evaluated against an activity that is more likely to produce change.

BARRIERS AND FACILITATORS

Good strategic planning is always cognizant of barriers and facilitators for change. Again, much can be learned from the research phase of the project. It is important for the durability planning group to take stock of past activities. What really worked? If a few activities that went

CHAPTER 8

Maintaining Preventive Health Efforts in Sub-Saharan Africa

AIDS in Tanzania

KNUT-INGE KLEPP
MELKIORY C. MASATU
PHILIP W. SETEL
GRO TH. LIE

Historically, culturally, and in terms of natural and human resources, the African continent represents an extremely rich and diverse part of the world. For historical reasons, including colonialism and economic exploitation, a large proportion of the people in sub-Saharan Africa do, however, live in extreme poverty today. It is estimated that the actual number of people in this region living in poverty will increase from 180 million in 1985 to 265 million by the year 2000 (World Bank, 1990). The health-related consequences of this poverty can clearly be read from international reports on morbidity and mortality (World Bank, 1993, 1997).

During the past decade, since the formulation of the World Health Organization (WHO) Health Promotion strategies (WHO, 1986), a large number of community-based health promotion projects have been initiated in Africa. Relatively few of these initiatives are, however, published and presented to a larger international audience. Furthermore, although a number of positive political events with clear health implications have taken place in Africa during the past decade (most noticeably, the end of apartheid in South Africa), this decade is also characterized by macrotrends with clear and profound negative health impacts throughout the African continent. These include

- A number of wars, causing, among other horrors, genocide, starvation, and large numbers of refugees, affecting the health and well-being of millions of people

- The introduction, in several countries, of neoliberal models of market-oriented economies, often dictated by international institutions such as the World Bank and the International Monetary Fund (IMF), resulting in increased economic inequity within the countries and a deterioration of social services provided by the governments, including education and health services (de la Barra, 1998)

- An increasing degree of urbanization, accompanied by the emergence of a number of "new" vulnerable groups, including the unemployed, commercial sex workers, homeless people, and street children

- The emergence of chronic disease patterns previously seen only in Western industrialized countries (cardiovascular diseases, cancer, and diabetes), traffic-related injuries and pollution, and infectious diseases (first of all the HIV/AIDS epidemic, but also malaria and reemerging epidemics of tuberculosis, cholera, and meningitis) (Ministry of Health & Adult Morbidity and Mortality Project Team, 1997)

These factors are all poverty related and have in themselves contributed to further impoverishment of large population groups. One result of this is seen in reported rates of malnutrition resulting in reduced growth (stunting among children under 5 years old). Although stunting decreased worldwide between 1980 and 1995, an increase (+0.13% per year) was observed in sub-Saharan Africa during this period (Administrative Committee on Coordination/Sub-Committee on Nutrition, United Nations, 1997). Thus, the actual number of children in this region affected by stunting increased by 62% during this period. There are, however, important differences among sub-Saharan African countries, and a number of countries made important progress with respect to stunting during the same period.

The African AIDS epidemic is a prime example of a poverty-driven epidemic. Due in large part to the lack of a health care system able to prevent and control other sexually transmitted diseases (Laga, Nzila, & Goeman, 1991), it is estimated that 20.8 million people in sub-Saharan Africa are HIV infected (7.4% of the adult population 15 to 49 years old) (United Nations AIDS Agency, 1997). In several sub-Saharan countries, large proportions of the active workforce have succumbed to AIDS, and this has had a devastating impact on the economic life of the communities; both children and the elderly have been left to care for themselves (Barnett & Blaikie, 1992).

With the exception of war (although a large number of refugees have come from neighboring Rwanda), all of the above factors apply to Tanzania, a country with an estimated 30 million people located in Eastern Africa just south of the equator. One of the world's poorest countries, Tanzania has recently made a peaceful transition from a one-party to a multiparty democracy.

In this chapter, we present some of our experiences from several years of implementing an AIDS control program in northeastern Tanzania. Since 1989, researchers and practitioners with backgrounds in social science, epidemiology, education, counseling, clinical medicine, and virology have joined forces in planning and implementing the National AIDS Control Program (NACP) in the Arusha and Kilimanjaro regions. In particular, we will focus on the planning, implementation, long-term impact, and sustainability of a school-based intervention initiative; a community counseling program; and a local, community-based, nongovernmental response to the HIV/AIDS epidemic.

AIDS in Tanzania

In Africa, Tanzania is among the countries having reported the largest number of AIDS cases. As of July 1996, a total of 88,667 cases had been reported to the World Health Organization (National AIDS Control Program [NACP], 1997). At the same time, the national authorities estimated the actual number of AIDS cases to be 450,000. A recent study in three districts of Tanzania furthermore revealed that HIV/AIDS is now the leading cause of death among adult (15 to 59 years) men and women in these areas (MOH/AMMP, 1997). The Kilimanjaro and Arusha regions rank as numbers 4 and 17 (out of 20 regions), with a cumulative AIDS case rate of 448.6 and 156.6 per 100,000 population, respectively, in 1996 (NACP, 1997). For both regions, this represents more than a doubling of the case rate just since 1993 (NACP, 1994).

In 1985, the Tanzanian government launched its first comprehensive AIDS control program (the Short Term Plan 1985-1987). This was followed by the First Medium Term Plan (MTP I) 1987-1991, which outlined a comprehensive HIV/AIDS prevention program under the Ministry of Health. It was organized through a National AIDS Control Program (NACP) located under the office of Preventive Services at the Ministry of Health. The Medium Term Plan II (MTP II) 1992-1996 represented a shift away from a vertical structure under MTP I, and it was based on the following principles (Swai, 1995):

- A multisectoral approach, including the involvement of nongovernmental organizations
- Decentralization of AIDS control efforts to the district levels
- Community mobilization
- Improved program management and coordination

During MTP II, the NACP still had the task of coordinating all AIDS prevention efforts, and it remained within the Ministry of Health.

MUTAN

In 1989, a contract was signed between the governments of Tanzania and Norway securing funding for a 5-year period (with a second 5-year period explicitly mentioned as a likely continuation) for implementation of the NACP in the Regions of Arusha and Kilimanjaro. The University of Dar es Salaam, Tanzania and the University of Bergen, Norway were asked to help implement the program and, in particular, to assist in design, methodological development, and evaluation of program activities. The contract for administrating the project was given to the University of Bergen. The local program was named the Tanzanian-Norwegian AIDS Control Project, or *Mradi wa UKIMWI wa Tanzania na Norway* (MUTAN).

An organizational structure was created, with the goal of integrating the activities within the existing health care structure and at the same time allowing for maximal flexibility to secure rapid action and effective use of resources earmarked for AIDS prevention (Figure 8.1). As can be seen from Figure 8.1, this structure clearly reflected the national AIDS policy at the time (MTP I), in

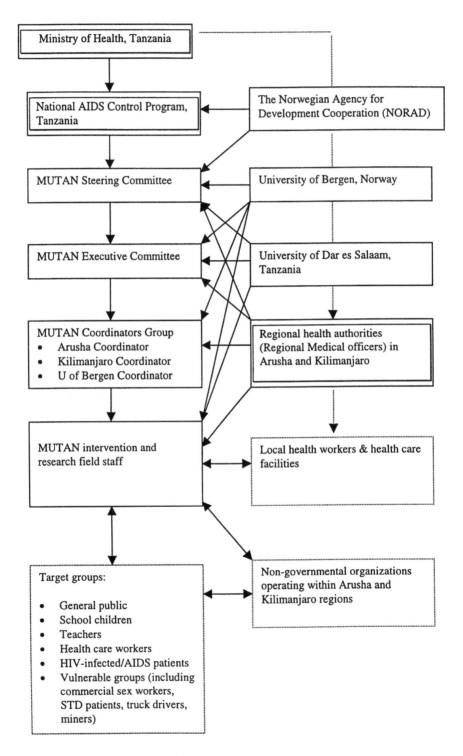

Figure 8.1. Organizational Chart for the MUTAN Project

that only the health sector was represented within the organization. The large majority of hired staff also represented the health sciences.

The MUTAN Steering Committee was chaired by the representative from the Tanzanian Ministry of Health and had representation from the donor agency (the Norwegian Agency for Development Cooperation [NORAD]) in addition to the local health authorities and the two universities. The committee met once a year; it was established to review the overall progress of the program, to assess and approve activity plans and budgets, and to provide directives for the executive committee. The executive committee consisted of two scientists (one from each university, at least one of whom had to be a social scientist), the regional medical officers, and the three project coordinators. The medical superintendent of the Kilimanjaro Christian Medical Center (KCMC) chaired this committee, which met regularly and provided guidelines for the three coordinators for their day-to-day running of the project (Bergsjø, 1996). Thus, the project had a very formal structure, was firmly embedded within the health sector, and there was no broader community representation within the project structure.

Target Communities

Tanzania consists of 20 regions, each again divided into a number of districts, divisions, wards, and villages. The smallest unit is the "10-cell," which consists of a cluster of about 10 households with an assigned leader. These geographical units reflect both the governmental administrative system and the party structure prior to the multiparty system.

The Arusha region is one of the most culturally complex areas in all of Africa. The region encompassed Bantu- and "Click"-speaking peoples who differ not only in language and culture but in economic adaptation and way of living. Many of the groups, such as the Maasai, adhere to a traditional way of life. The Kilimanjaro region, however, is far more homogenous ethnically, with the Chagga being the largest group. Other factors that add to the heterogeneity of Arusha and Kilimanjaro are lifestyle differences between urban and rural areas and a growing economic differentiation that is particularly visible in the urban centers.

Overall, the majority of the population in the two regions consists of peasant farmers whose production is oriented primarily toward their own subsistence. Most of them are, nonetheless, dependent upon a market for produce sales and cash. Some 20% live in urban and semiurban areas, and a large portion of these survive on temporary jobs and businesses. In 1988, the total population in the area was close to 2.5 million, divided almost equally between the two regions. Because Kilimanjaro is much smaller in area, its population density is much higher than that of Arusha: 83 and 16 persons per square kilometer, respectively (Bureau of Statistics [Tanzania], 1990). The regional centers Arusha and Moshi are rapidly expanding urban areas.

In the late 1970s and early 1980s, Tanzania suffered an economic crisis from which it has taken more than a decade to emerge (Sarris & Tinios, 1995). The collapse was brought about by a combination of internal and external forces, including the oil crisis, poor fiscal policy and planning, and a spiraling debt burden. It culminated in the adoption of an IMF and World Bank-brokered Economic Structural Adjustment Program that substantially curtailed public sector expenditures, particularly in health. Between 1979 and 1982, the average retail price index for goods and services used by urban populations doubled (Cheru, 1989). By the late 1980s, workers were earning 65% less in real wages compared to what they had made in the mid-1970s, and consumer prices had risen tenfold (Tripp, 1989). A strict reliance on agricultural production, formal sector, or public sector employment became unsupportable, the "informal sector"[1] exploded, and women and young people entered the cash economy in unprecedented numbers. This social and economic upheaval and uncertainty in Tanzania was the environment into which AIDS emerged in the early to mid-1980s.

At the start of the MUTAN project, there was, clearly, a paucity of information regarding local HIV/AIDS-related knowledge, beliefs, and practices, as well as cultural norms and socio-economic factors that might put people at increased risk for HIV infection. Prior to designing the intervention programs, a number of studies were therefore conducted to investigate potential risk factors and factors that might facilitate program implementation within various population groups. These epidemiological (Klouman, Masenga, Klepp, et al., 1997; Lugoe, Klepp, Rise, Skutle, & Biswalo, 1995; Lugoe, Klepp, & Skutle, 1996; Mnyika, Klepp, Kvåle, Nilssen, et al., 1994; Mnyika, Klepp, Kvåle, Schreiner, & Seha, 1995; Ndeki, Klepp, Seha, & Leshabari, 1994; Ngomuo, Klepp, Rise, & Mnyika, 1995) and social anthropological (Blystad, 1995; Haram, 1995; Heguye, 1995; Setel, 1995b, 1997; Talle, 1995a, 1995b) studies greatly increased our understanding of what factors make young people particularly vulnerable to the AIDS epidemic. The studies were, however, less effective than intended in guiding the intervention programs, mainly because the results were not available in time (due to delayed research clearance[2] and time-consuming data analysis). Thus, the community analyses conducted prior to program design relied, to a large extent, on the local knowledge and experience of the Tanzanian project staff.

HIV/AIDS Prevention Efforts in Arusha and Kilimanjaro

The overall objective of the NACP was to implement a comprehensive HIV/AIDS control program (Swai, 1995), including strategies to

- Prevent sexual transmission of HIV
- Prevent transmission through blood, blood products, and skin-piercing activities
- Reduce transmission from mother to child
- Provide support for HIV-infected people with and without AIDS
- Provide health care for these people
- Promote action to reduce the social and economic consequences of the HIV/AIDS epidemic

The MUTAN project, responsible for these NACP strategies in Arusha and Kilimanjaro, designed a number of programs to reach the general public, as well as important target groups. Informed consent had to be obtained from local administrative and political leaders at all levels prior to implementing any of the prevention activities, including recruitment of other community members to take part in planning or implementation of programs. This gave a necessary and important opportunity for providing information to the local leadership, building alliances, and securing local support. To obtain local leaders' support, project staff frequently had to listen to them express the concerns and needs of their communities. As a result, we learned that HIV/AIDS often was not perceived as the most critical health issue, and that other problems, such as clean drinking water, had to be addressed before the HIV/AIDS work could proceed. An overview of target groups and intervention strategies is presented in Table 8.1. Detailed presentations of the various intervention components and evaluation results have been presented elsewhere (Bergsjø, Olomi, Talle, & Klepp, 1995; Klepp, Ndeki, Seha, et al., 1994; Klepp, Msuya, Lyimo, & Bergsjø, 1995; Klouman, Masenga, Sam, & Lauwo, 1995; Lie, Biswalo, & Klepp, 1995; Mnyika, Klepp, Ole-Kingóri, & Seha, 1995; Mollel, Olomi, Mwanga, & Mongi, 1995).

In this chapter, we have chosen to focus on three initiatives, illustrating different strategies for mobilizing local community resources in the fight against the HIV/AIDS epidemic. These are: a school-based educational program targeting students in elementary schools, a community counseling approach pilot-tested in a village in Arusha region, and the formation and work by a women's group against AIDS in Kilimanjaro.

THE NGAO SCHOOL PROGRAM

The majority of young people in Tanzania complete 7 years of primary school, but few have the opportunity for further schooling. Primary schools, especially the 6th and 7th grades (when most pupils are 13 to 15 years old), in which a large number of pupils state that they are sexually active (Ndeki, Klepp, & Mliga, 1994), therefore constitute an important arena for HIV prevention work. We prepared and tested a curriculum that provided teachers with opportunities to adapt their lessons to more closely fit local norms and traditions. A number of activities, although school-based, were designed to actively involve other community members, including health care workers, parents, and community leaders.

The program was named *Ngao*, meaning "shield," an often-used symbol in Tanzania and in particular among the ethnic Maasai. The Ngao is a symbol indicating that young people should be able to protect themselves from HIV infection. The purpose of the Ngao program was to help pupils make informed decisions about how to avoid AIDS-related risk behaviors. To achieve this goal, the following specific objectives were put forth:

- Increase children's awareness of AIDS and its magnitude and severity
- Increase their knowledge about HIV/AIDS, its transmission, and appropriate preventive measures
- Create more positive attitudes about socializing with and caring for people with AIDS
- Foster attitudes and subjective norms that reduce the intention to engage in and actual involvement with HIV risk-related behaviors
- Teach social skills that may increase children's abilities to avoid high-risk situations

Due to the ethnic and cultural variety within the Arusha and Kilimanjaro regions, as well as the large urban-rural differences, the educational materials were designed so that teachers could modify them according to the specific norms and attitudes of their own local community. Prior to writing the school curriculum, the AIDS education team conducted a literature search, reviewing

TABLE 8.1 Target Groups and Intervention Strategies Employed as Part of the National AIDS Control Program Implemented by MUTAN in the Arusha and Kilimanjaro Regions

Target Groups	Intervention Strategies
General public	*Mass media:* Weekly radio programs (15 min) broadcast nationally. Addressed themes related to HIV/AIDS prevention and counseling and treatment of AIDS patients. Responded to questions raised by listeners.
	Information centers: Located in Arusha and Moshi; provided information, condoms, and counseling services to the public.
	Public meetings: Open, outdoor HIV/AIDS education meetings at marketplaces and in conjunction with the Information Centers.
	STD clinics: Specially staffed and equipped clinics in Arusha and Moshi municipalities providing STD treatment and preventive services.
	Nongovernmental organizations: Joint meetings for religious groups and other organizations for information exchange, policy discussions, and coordination of efforts.
	Condom promotion: Condoms were handed out free of charge through hotels, health care facilities, the Information Centers, and in connection with all HIV/AIDS surveys.
Community leaders	*HIV/AIDS courses:* 5- to 10-day intensive courses for party secretaries, village leaders, and leaders of youth and women's organizations; the goal was to give them a thorough introduction to HIV/AIDS-related issues.
Teachers	*Health education:* Short courses providing information on HIV/AIDS transmission and prevention and effective educational methods.
Schoolchildren	*School-based education (Ngao):* Participatory and behavior-focused educational program for students in Standards 6 and 7; taught by teachers with assistance from local health care workers.
Health care workers	*STD training:* Training in how to detect, treat, and prevent STDs offered at local health care facilities and at the STD clinics in Arusha and Moshi.
	Counseling: Training in how to provide pre- and posttest counseling for AIDS patients and patients taking an HIV test.
	Health education: Short courses providing information on HIV/AIDS transmission and prevention and appropriate care.
	Blood screening: Training in how to secure safe blood transfusions and reporting of data to the NACP.
People with HIV or AIDS	*Counseling:* Trained counselors provided in-hospital and home-based follow-up counseling services.
	Home care: Several religious groups and hospital-based counselors conducted home visits, providing care and counseling services.
Bar workers, truck drivers, and miners	*Peer education:* Commercial sex workers in communities regarded as high HIV-transmission areas were trained as peer leaders, providing information and condoms to other commercial sex workers, truck drivers, and miners (in high HIV-transmission communities)
	STD clinics: The two established STD clinics would specifically target perceived vulnerable groups such as bar workers and other commercial sex workers.

available educational material produced by others, including the African Medical and Research Foundation (AMREF), the Red Cross, and the National AIDS Control Programs in Tanzania and in neighboring countries. Furthermore, we consulted with local teachers, health workers, and the social anthropologists conducting AIDS-related research in the two regions. A theoretical framework guided by the Theory of Reasoned Action (Fishbein & Middlestadt, 1989) and by Social Cognitive Theory (Bandura, 1992) was employed to identify the important factors believed to influence the onset of high-risk behaviors (Klepp, Ndeki, Thuen, Leshabari, & Seha, 1996).

A teacher's manual and a booklet for pupils to take home were produced. The materials were written in English by project health educators, then translated to Swahili, the official language used in primary schools. A minimum of two teachers and one local health worker were invited from each participating school to attend a 1-week training workshop. Following this workshop, the program was implemented over the course of a 2- to 3-month period, averaging about 25 to 30 school hours per class.

Rather than relying on audiovisual equipment not readily available throughout the regions (most schools lack electricity), classroom activities that could be implemented with a minimum of resources were emphasized. Traditional didactic methods of teaching were used for information dissemination, but teachers also received training in how to use more interactive techniques. Thus, teachers were encouraged to let the pupils engage in group discussions and to write and perform their own role plays, songs, and poems in response to the information presented. Teachers also received training in how they could select and train certain pupils who were respected and liked by other pupils to be peer leaders. These pupils were trained in how to conduct small group discussions and role-play activities and how to summarize and report group findings to the class. Topics for the group discussions included "What puts young people in our society at risk for becoming HIV infected?" and "What can people our age do to avoid high-risk situations?" To support this participatory learning, instructional materials such as chalkboards, visual aids (such as posters and drawings), and pamphlets were used. Also, a number of activities were designed to increase communication with parents and other community members regarding AIDS. Such activities included interviews with parents and with other family members and friends and panel discussions at schools to which community elders, religious leaders, and parents were invited to discuss how the community could take action against AIDS. These activities are summarized in Table 8.2.

The results from the evaluation of this program have been presented in detail elsewhere (Klepp, Ndeki, Leshabari, Hannan, & Lyimo, 1997; Klepp, Ndeki, Seha, et al., 1994). In short, after 12 months, significant effects favoring the intervention group were observed for exposure to AIDS information and communication, AIDS knowledge, attitudes toward people with AIDS, subjective norms toward having sexual intercourse, and behavioral intention. A consistent, positive, but non-statistically-significant trend was seen for attitudes toward having sexual intercourse and onset of sexual intercourse during the past year (7% vs. 17%). It was concluded that it is feasible and effective to train local teachers and health workers to provide HIV/AIDS education to Tanzanian primary school children (Klepp, Ndeki, Leshabari, et al., 1997).

Sustainability

The program was implemented in 1992. Following the 12-month evaluation, teachers and health workers at the comparison schools were trained in how to implement the program. Five years later (in 1997), former MUTAN researchers conducted a follow-up study among same-age

TABLE 8.2 Ngao School-Based HIV/AIDS Education Program Activities

---

- Teachers and local health workers provided factual information regarding HIV transmission and AIDS. Specific top-ics included
  - What is AIDS? What causes this disease? How severe is it?
  - What is the extent of the problem in our region and in Tanzania?
  - How is HIV transmitted? How is it not transmitted?
  - What are the signs and symptoms of an HIV-infected person and of an AIDS patient?
  - How can we care for and support someone with the HIV virus or with AIDS?
- Pupils made their own posters depicting their perceptions of HIV risk factors and wrote and performed songs and po-etry about the danger of AIDS and how children their own age could protect themselves.
- Pupils worked in small groups, discussing how people are exposed to HIV risk and what they themselves could do to reduce such risk. When appropriate, brainstorming and group discussions were conducted for boys and girls sepa-rately. Peer leaders helped facilitate group discussions, which focused on questions such as
  - What can people our age do to prevent the spread of HIV?
  - What do other people in our community (our friends, parents, teachers, religious leaders, elders, health workers) think about people our age drinking alcohol? being sexually active?
  - What are our attitudes towards HIV-infected people? Toward being sexually active?
- Pupils wrote and performed role plays in which they tried to convince each other to avoid HIV risk behaviors or prac-tice refusal skills relating to sexual behavior. They also created and performed elaborate plays in which they wore their traditional clothes and portrayed how AIDS could be dealt with in their community.
- The plays, role plays, poetry, and songs were performed outdoors in front of younger pupils attending the school. In this way, the program had the potential to educate these younger children.
- Community elders, religious leaders, and parents were invited to participate in panel discussions at schools to discuss how their community could take action against AIDS.
- All pupils received a T-shirt with the Ngao symbol. This increased the visibility of the program and helped foster in-creased communication regarding AIDS.

---

pupils attending the same schools. Preliminary results from this survey indicate that pupils attending the original intervention schools had slightly better knowledge levels but that there were no differences in terms of attitudes toward people with AIDS or having had their sexual debut compared to pupils attending the comparison schools. Overall, pupils in 1997 did not express more positive attitudes toward people with AIDS than did pupils at the 1992 baseline survey.

COMMUNITY COUNSELING

By the late 1980s, health personnel throughout the Arusha and Kilimanjaro regions were seeing AIDS patients. How to comfort and support these patients in the absence of an effective treatment was the number one question asked by health personnel at the inception of MUTAN. Training health personnel in how to provide counseling services was therefore one of the first initiatives taken by MUTAN (Lie, Biswalo, & Klepp,1995). Having established these services at the major hospitals, MUTAN embarked on developing and testing a model for HIV/AIDS community counseling. The model was pilot-tested in a village in the Arusha region located along the main road approximately 30 km from Arusha town. The objectives of this counseling approach were to prevent further spread of HIV in the village, fight the stigma of AIDS, and assist people with HIV/AIDS in the village (Lie & Biswalo, 1995). This was attempted through

- providing HIV/AIDS education for community members at large;
- influencing community leaders and public policy;
- providing outreach services for vulnerable clients; and
- advocating the rights of the clients.

Eight people, trusted and respected in their village, able to deal with sensitive issues and solve problems, and aware of resources within their own community were selected by the village chairman to serve as lay counselors (the selection criteria were set by the project staff). These lay counselors (three men and five women) differed with regard to age, ethnic group, religion, level of education, and occupation. They were trained and supervised by senior MUTAN counselors.

The Community Analysis

A community analysis was conducted as a basis for the plan of action, and it also served as a point of departure for monitoring changes and evaluating effects. The analysis was conducted by the lay counselors themselves and included basic demographic and socioeconomic data, village institutions, organizations and group structures, normative structures, and behavior patterns of relevance to HIV/AIDS problems. The lay counselors received training in how to conduct the analysis and followed strict ethical guidelines for the collection and use of this information. Comprehensive findings from this community analysis are presented elsewhere (Lie & Biswalo, 1995).

To give a sense of some of the challenges of and resources available for conducting community-based work on a village level, a brief presentation of this information is included here.

The village had a total of 2,647 inhabitants, of whom 1,052 were below the age of 15. It consisted of 21 10-cells, and 20 ethnic groups were represented in the village. Single, unmarried people constituted approximately 40% of the adult population. About 10% of the adult population lived in traditional extended family systems, 20% lived in so-called nuclear families (mother, father, and children), and as many as 30% of the adults were single parents.

The village had no primary or secondary school. The children had to walk long distances to neighboring villages for education. The village also had no public health care facility. There was one private dispensary in the village and a public dispensary close by. Several traditional healers practiced in the village. Villagers were predominantly Christian and Moslem, and religious groups such as women's groups and choirs played a significant role in the everyday life of the community.

The local soccer team also had an important position in the community, attracting large numbers of spectators to its games. The team members were, furthermore, popular role models among boys and young men. The village had a high number of retail shops, beer and soda bars, and *pombe* (local brew) shops, which were open daily from 9 a.m. to midnight. There were also several authorized and nonauthorized guesthouses and hotels nearby, and a busy marketplace. The unemployment rate was extremely high in the village, and many relied on seasonal agricultural work. Illicit production of local brews and liquor and, for women, commercial sex work were common strategies for securing the daily food. The average adult income was estimated at TAS 2,000 per month (US$6 to $7 a month in 1993).

In 1992, the village inhabitants, traditional healers, and local health workers all reported AIDS not to be a common health problem in this village. People furthermore associated AIDS with shame and misbehavior, and many of those interviewed said they would not be willing to care for AIDS patients, blaming the AIDS patients themselves for their misfortune. At the time there were actually five AIDS patients receiving follow-up counseling in the village. None of them dared to be open about the disease, as they feared rejection. A large HIV screening and interview survey, conducted earlier the same year, had found 2% of the villagers (15 to 54 years old) to be HIV-positive (Mnyika, Klepp, Kvåle, Nilssen, et al., 1994). These survey data had also indicated that a high proportion of the villagers had multiple sexual partners. This was in contrast to the restrictive sexual norms expressed in interviews to the lay counselors. Thus, there seemed to be considerable discrepancy between expressed norms and actual sexual behavior.

Plan of Action
and Implementation

The counselors made a commitment to meet at least once a week to plan and report on their work. Based on their analysis, they decided to focus on two target groups: (a) members of the soccer team and (b) young unmarried and unemployed women. Members of the soccer team were popular role models but were also among those who reported changing sexual partners most frequently. The counselors focused on the soccer team as a group, trying to alter the group's sexual behavior norms and foster a collective commitment to reduce risky sexual behavior.

The young unmarried and unemployed women were seen as a vulnerable group for entering commercial sex work or becoming pregnant at a young age. The young women were more difficult to reach as a group, and in order not to stigmatize them, it was determined to conduct public HIV/AIDS education meetings at the 10-cell level.

To the surprise of the counselors, the villagers were very open about discussing sexuality. Those who attended the public meetings agreed to motivate other family members and neighbors to come as well, and gradually the attendance rate grew. The meetings became useful forums for discussing fear and misconceptions held by villagers. One outcome of these meetings was the decision that villagers should be able to get condoms from the female counselors (to increase access to condoms, particularly for the young women). Another outcome was that the young women decided to start small businesses (to become self-employed), and they set out to make specific plans. Finally, these meetings seemed to start a process that made it possible for people to discuss HIV/AIDS in various settings, including the marketplace, bars, churches, and mosques. Some of the church choirs wrote and performed AIDS education songs, and local business owners came to the counselors and asked for AIDS education to be given to their employees. It was also requested that the younger children (including school-age children 13 to 14 years old) should receive AIDS education.

The AIDS patients in the village continued to receive home-visits from the hospital counselors. Some of these patients were afraid that their neighbors might understand the nature of their illness as they learned more about AIDS. The patients were not convinced that they would be accepted, having heard people say that AIDS patients should be left to themselves and not burden the community. However, some had noticed a more caring attitude. In spite of some progress, the reality of a caring community was still a future vision.

anthropological studies from around Africa, however, suggest that playing the "culture card" can too easily trump a more reasoned consideration of the overriding influences of poverty and social insecurity (Jochelson, 1991; Packard & Epstein, 1991; Schoepf, 1988). Tanzania is one of the poorest countries in the world. The information presented in this chapter demonstrates how poverty at the local level is translated into personal risk for HIV infection and is a critical barrier to sustained health promotion efforts at a local level. Furthermore, lack of economic resources in the public sector creates serious barriers to be overcome if health promotion efforts are to be truly effective; fully one third of the Tanzanian national budget is spent on debt servicing, but barely a third of that amount is allocated to health and education combined.

The MUTAN experience illustrates the vulnerability of health promotion efforts dependent upon foreign donors. As the first phase of the project (1989-1994) ended, it took 2 years before the Norwegian Agency for Development Cooperation (NORAD) decided to renew the contract, this time without the MUTAN structure. In an effort to strengthen the governmental structures in Tanzania, money was given directly to NACP. A prerequisite for this donation was that MUTAN be dissolved, as NORAD felt it had become too much of a parallel structure to the Tanzanian governmental bureaucracy. During this 2-year lag period, key staff assumed other positions, and key activities at a local level came to a halt. Thus, although important policy changes regarding national HIV/AIDS prevention work took place (note the shift from MTP I to MTP II), policy changes at the donor level (in this case the Norwegian government) play a profound and often unpredictable role in local attempts to sustain health promotion efforts in resource-poor settings.

MUTAN managed to become an effective organization, partly imbedded within the governmental structure but at the same time with an independent mode of operation, almost like a local version of the NACP itself. This is evident from the number of activities designed and pilot-tested and the wealth of information made available through this project. Furthermore, it was demonstrated that the theoretical foundation for school- and community-based interventions largely developed in Western societies could be modified and adapted successfully to guide local health promotion efforts also in an East African setting.

MUTAN never managed, however, to create a comprehensive community-based strategy across the two regions. Thus, although the activities listed in Table 8.1 were implemented within the two regions, no single community was exposed to all of them. The three examples provided in this chapter, the schools program, the community counseling approach, and the formation of a women's group against AIDS, illustrate this problem. These activities took place in different communities, and there was no system in place for securing large dissemination of program components or a comprehensive strategy as soon as the pilot work had been successfully completed. Furthermore, no systematic attempt to include community representation (lay representation or professional representation from sectors other than the health sector) was built into the MUTAN organization across the two regions.

A comprehensive community-based strategy requires that some basic information and intervention tools be in place. This was largely the case in Arusha and Kilimanjaro by the mid-1990s when NORAD funding was disrupted. Why, then, was the NACP local governmental structure not able to use this information and continue the work within the framework provided by MTP II? The lack of effective communication is a key factor to understanding the disruption that occurred. Mass media coverage is poor and almost nonexistent in the rural areas. Thus there are no inexpensive and effective ways of rapidly disseminating information to large population groups. The stigma still attached to HIV/AIDS, as evident from the school survey and the village work, will continue, as rumors and misconceptions are spread as effectively as are health education messages. No celebrity or high-status individuals with HIV, no local Magic Johnson, emerged as a focal point for AIDS activism. Furthermore, communication among rural and centrally located health care workers, teachers, or NGO representatives has been hampered by an expensive or poorly functioning telephone system, poor roads, and the scarcity of vehicles. In such conditions, conveying a message or conducting a meeting with a colleague just a few kilometers outside of town becomes a major event that can take a day just in terms of travel time. Thus, communication becomes extremely costly and labor intensive, creating major barriers having to be faced in all phases of a health promotion program implemented within a relatively small geographical area.

As Tanzania takes on the implementation of the current MTP III, the time seems ripe to embark on a large-scale dissemination of a comprehensive approach, implementing the various strategies (developed during MUTAN as well as elsewhere over the past decade) in a systematic fashion and embedded within a community-based approach. Although such an approach would rely on local resources, a minimum of support has to be available through the public sectors as well as through local and national NGOs. Finally, health promotion efforts in resource-poor settings in general, and HIV/AIDS prevention in particular, require a long-term commitment from all actors involved.

Notes

1. The informal sector consists of unregistered petty traders and small-business men and women.

2. Research clearance for AIDS-related research is given by the National AIDS Control Program. This review process was not firmly established at the time, and the delay was primarily caused by bureaucratic incapability.

3. More information about KIWAKKUKI, including its annual reports, can be obtained from its treasurer, Janet Lefroy, at lefroy@form-net.com.

9

Asia and Western Pacific Approaches to Health Promotion

Current Opportunities and Programs

RHONDA GALBALLY

BRIDGET H.-H. HSU-HAGE

CHRIS BORTHWICK

Social and Political Background

The Asia and Western Pacific region is perhaps the most heterogeneous of any of the world's regions. It includes 29 states that range in size from islands of 260 square kilometers to continents of $7\frac{1}{2}$ million, from thousands of people to more than a billion, from $650 per capita GDP to $23,000, from $3 per capita health expenditure to $1,538, from life expectancies of 50 years to 80. Cultures, political systems, religions, climates, and lifestyles are very different. Approaches to health promotion in this region thus arise from different contexts to serve different needs.[1]

Social, Cultural, and Political Systems

Given the extent of these differences between societies in the region, no single approach to health promotion would be feasible. The post–World War II period saw rapid political transformations among many nations in the region. Political systems today range from communist governments to monarchies and from liberal democracies to authoritarian regimes, with a large number of nations operating under capitalist economic systems with elected governments that nonetheless believe in a high degree of government involvement in the direction of economic, social, cultural, and political life. The region's cultures range from modernized Confucianism to Western individualism. Nations such as Malaysia and Singapore favor an Asian way that stresses order, consensus, discipline, family values, filial loyalty, and deference to authority. This emphasis on community-level rather than individually focused action is in harmony with the move away from the individual behavior change model of the Western world. Western concepts of empowerment, however, may in Asia be interpreted and applied in such a way as to comply with the prevailing societal expectation.

Literacy

The importance of sectors other than the health sector to population health status has been better appreciated in the region following the World Bank's (1993) stress on the connection between literacy rates and maternal and child health, which demonstrated that the most important factor in reducing perinatal mortality rates was the purely educational intervention of raising female literacy rates. Leaving aside Cambodia, whose years of warfare make it a special case, literacy rates in the region range from 99% in Japan to 57% in Laos. All nations in the region are committed to universal education, mostly directed toward economic growth and often restrained by considerations of finance, distance and terrain, and poverty.

Economic Growth

Many nations in the Asia-Pacific region have experienced rapid economic growth (in some cases from an extremely low base). This has improved basic health status, such as the incidence of malnutrition, and has made possible increased spending on primary health. It has also, however, involved increased urbanization and increased environmental degradation, and although this is not yet a general constraint on population health, it will undoubtedly in the future cause major problems in the area of noncommunicable diseases. The choking smog that bathed Kuala Lumpur for several months in 1997, caused by forests burning in Indonesian Borneo, is an undeniable indication that the ecological problems of the region are beginning to press on the determinants of health. Economically, too, the rampant growth that has in much of Asia created both the threats to health and the resources to address them has been shown to be vulnerable to sudden reversals, and the effects of this on health and health promotion programs have yet to be felt.

Health Issues

HEALTH INDICATORS

Mortality rates in the region have fallen precipitously since the war, with increased prosperity and improved public health; these gains may have plateaued, however, and further progress may become more difficult. The World Bank has pioneered the concept of the DALY, or disability adjusted life year (Murray, 1997), which has had the particular advantage of drawing attention to the health impact of conditions like mental illness that have comparatively little effect on mortality statistics but nonetheless represent a large proportion of national morbidity.

The measurement of health is also complicated in this region by the effects of cultural and ethnic differences. For example, measurement of intermediate indicators concerned with food and nutrition such as obesity, cholesterol levels, and dietary patterns across the region presents some difficulties, in that these indicators have not in general been adjusted to take account of the different body types of regional populations. The lack of differential epidemiological studies in each of the nations of the region has resulted in adoption of program approaches based on criteria identified by studies of Western populations. Measures of obesity or other risk indicators need be recalibrated to reflect the true differences of risk prevalence in the region. The health significance of body mass index (a measure of body fatness), for example, cannot be expected to be identical in Samoans, Australians, and Chinese. Social epidemiology, too, will need to be re-created to incorporate indicators that are meaningful for different cultures, and there is a need for further research on quality-of-life measures that are not culturally confounded.

CHANGING DISEASE PATTERNS

The problems faced by peoples of the region also fall at different points along the much-discussed epidemiological transition from a predominance in mortality and morbidity statistics of acute infectious diseases to one with increasing rates of chronic cardiovascular and cerebrovascular diseases and cancers. In some nations, such as Australia and New Zealand, infectious diseases have been largely controlled, and the so-called lifestyle diseases are the main concern. In other nations in the region, improvements in infectious disease rates have not yet eliminated the threat to health from malnutrition, respiratory diseases, tuberculosis, hepatitis, and other infections, while at the same time increasing rates of urbanization, an increasingly prosperous middle class, and changing age profiles have increased the rates of noncommunicable disease and mental illness.

In China, for example, heart disease has risen from the fifth most common cause of death to the first, and heart disease deaths have risen from 6.6% to 23% of deaths. The rate of stroke in urban areas has doubled. The most common causes of premature death are blood pressure and chronic lung disease. Road trauma deaths and injuries are also rising sharply. The increased reach of immunization and the development of antibiotics and antituberculosis drugs have dramatically decreased the mortality rate from infectious diseases since World War II. These new problems have turned the spotlight on the changes in the approaches to health promotion that have accompanied the changes in the disease burden in Western nations.

Traditional public health approaches such as sanitation and mass immunization programs are essential to maintain the basic health of the population, and their importance is everywhere recognized in the region (although not all nations put the necessary resources behind these programs: Australia's immunization rates are particularly low). It is also increasingly recognized that the prevention of noncommunicable and communicable lifestyle diseases (HIV/AIDS) depends crucially on behavior change, social factors, and environmental supports, and that greater emphasis must thus be placed on social and cultural factors as they affect health status. Socially oriented approaches to health promotion focusing on community empowerment have, to date, been influential mainly in Australia and New Zealand, although developments along these lines are now under way in several Asia-Pacific nations.

CHANGING PATTERNS OF CONSUMPTION

The newer health problems of the Asia-Pacific region are associated with the disruption to traditional practices arising out of the close integration of Asian economies into a global system of production and consumption. Tobacco, for example, represents only the most damaging end of a drive to shift from traditional social patterns to full participation in a Westernized, consumption-driven society. The upheavals in traditional social relationships that this transformation involves have their own effects on health through a loss of cultural coherence and a rise in personal insecurity.

Food and Nutrition

Food- and nutrition-related health issues will continue to command the attention of nations in the region, moving from solving the basic need of food and the problem of malnutrition in some areas to finding a solution for the explosion of overnutrition associated with the region's rapid and widespread economic growth. This growth has brought with it increased purchasing power, including food and health, to the people of the region. The phenomenon of rapid urbanization and the globalization in trade and financial markets all help further diminish the geographic boundary of traditional food supply, leaving the region faced with new threats such as food security, as well as new nutrition challenges typified by the presence of both undernutrition and overnutrition within many nations and within subgroups of those nations.

There are also issues related to particular national diets. In Japan, alterations in health practices, such as decreasing the intake of salty foods and strict management of hypertension, have resulted in important decreases in the mortality rate from cerebrovascular diseases, especially from cerebral hemorrhage (Sakata & Moriyama, 1990). As Western foods and cooking styles become more accepted and more widespread, however, the Japanese protection from many of the West's problems has also diminished, and such diseases as bladder and colon cancer are on the rise.

Tobacco

The rise in smoking rates in Asia has also shifted the health risk patterns. As cigarettes were very scarce in Japan after the war, Japanese men started smoking in rapidly increasing numbers only in the 1950s and 1960s. The 20- to 30-year lag curve between starting smoking and developing health problems means that the mortality statistics are just catching up, and lung cancer is now an important and increasing cause of death in Japan. It has been since 1993 the leading cause of cancer deaths among Japanese men in 1993, at 29%. As female smoking rates are still low, only 8% of female cancer deaths involve lung cancer. In 1995, the World Health Organization (WHO) estimated that tobacco would cause 14% of all deaths (20% male, 8% female), and that proportion is still increasing among both males and females (Chen, Xu, Collins, Li, & Peto, 1997).

The increasing reach of multinational corporations and Western advertising images, coupled with increasing prosperity, has now resulted in an explosion of smoking rates across the Western Pacific region. After South Korea opened up its cigarette market to U.S. companies in 1988, smoking rates among male Korean teenagers jumped from 18.4% to 29.8% in a single year, while the rate among young females more than quintupled, from 1.6% to 8.7%.

Australia has tight regulations on tobacco advertising, with an almost complete ban on all cigarette advertising in any format other than point of sale. Thailand has also recently tightened regulations on cigarette advertising.[2] Vietnam has strict regulations on the amount of Western material allowed in the country—Western magazine ads and outdoor billboards, for example, were removed in a recent crackdown on Western products—but the ever-increasing pressures of globalization mean that this is likely to be of only short-term advantage to the antitobacco movement.

In Indonesia, rising per capita income has led to higher smoking rates. Cigarette advertising is currently allowed on Indonesian TV as long as cigarette packs and smoking scenes are not shown. The government still sees tobacco as a revenue source, tobacco interests have strong political links, and the government has not yet moved to take strong steps to discourage the habit. Indonesian preferences for clove-scented kreteks over imported cigarettes provides some barrier to internationalization but may also embed tobacco use more deeply into the nation's economy, culture, and politics. In Singapore, by contrast, smoking is vigorously discouraged: Advertising has been banned since 1971 (although there have been problems with cross-border leakage of the less-regulated Malaysian media), smoking is banned in most public venues, tobacco sponsorship of sport is banned, and restrictions are placed on tar levels. Korea has met the constant pressure on health funding by setting up a levy on tobacco sales to fund health promotion, and several nations in the region are now considering similar arrangements.

ECONOMIC GROWTH AND WORKPLACE HEALTH

Increasing urbanization and industrialization in the countries of the region have created new stresses on health in the workplace environment. Workplace health promotion has made its greatest impact in those countries with a tradition of strong union coverage and lifetime employment. Health promotion in Japan, for example, has had its greatest success in the field of occupational health, with health guidance, fitness, and nutrition education programs. In line with the Japanese tradition of company cohesiveness, environmental measures such as zoning of smoking areas are generally favored over such individually directed measures such as smoking cessation programs (Muto et al., 1996). It is also true that occupational health measures are not often linked with organizational change. WHO is, however, developing guidelines for the development of health-promoting workplaces across the region that will not only stress accident prevention but also cover such organizational factors as the nature of work, workload, the distribution of power and control, autonomy, coherence, the division of labor, managment ethos and style, and company communication systems, all of which contribute significantly to the health of the workplace.

The Influence of International Agencies

In more general terms, the Asia-Pacific region has been greatly influenced by the work of WHO in providing "a credible environment for advocacy" (Buasai, 1997, p. 18). In this region, however, the immense challenges of poverty and disease have meant that WHO's main efforts have until now necessarily been largely centered around medical and public health initiatives rather than the social directions of the Ottowa charter. WHO's material acknowledges the wider picture.

> A wide range of factors external to the individual, such as urbanization, industrializa-
> tion, migration, and environmental changes in the course of development affect
> individual health. The problems involved must be tackled successfully in support of
> individuals' efforts to better their own health. (Han & Erben, 1993, p. 36)

Its practice, however, is largely restricted to support for interventions directed at informing and educating individuals in lifestyle health issues, approaches that have in the West been shown to have only limited success (Winkleby, Taylor, Jatulis, & Fortmann, 1996).

The World Bank's (1993) view that investment in health and in disease prevention makes an appreciable contribution to economic growth has also played an important role; health ministries are rarely as influential in government policymaking as finance ministries, and where (as in Thailand) these can be persuaded of the importance of health promotion, then support for organizational infrastructure is more likely.

Health Promotion Approaches and Practices

The historical development from public health to health promotion approaches is illustrated by examples from the region. In Australia, as in much of the West, traditional public health based on state responsibility for water, sewage, and immunization developed from the 1950s to include mass media campaigns targeting the so-called lifestyle diseases. These campaigns were largely individu- ally focused and relied on individuals to take responsibility for their own health. These methods were, unfortunately, often transferred without modification to Asian environments, becoming accepted there just as their limitations were becoming apparent in the West. By contrast, the "new public health" approaches focus on the community and environmental level as essential for the achievement of individual lifestyle behavioral modification. In countries where basic health needs such as peace, shelter, education, food, income, respect for human rights, and equity remain a problem, health promotion continues to be challenged and tested.

In several places, special taxes are being levied on tobacco products to raise money for health promotion. The logic of this action is clear when the impact of tobacco on health and its human and financial costs are calculated. It is a strategy that is being employed in the Republic of Korea, in New Zealand, in several states in Australia and the United States of America, and it is currently under consideration in Canada, France, Fiji, and Thailand.

Approaches that work in one country cannot be expected to be transferable without major cultural adjustment. In this region, where the degree of health development varies so greatly, there

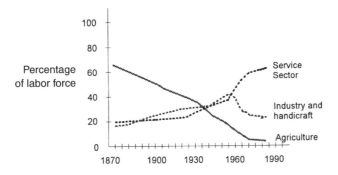

Figure 10.1. Occupational Development in Sweden, 1870–1990

travel, and vacations. In Norway, less than 15% of the average family income is now spent on food, compared with 40% 40 years ago (Central Bureau of Statistics, Norway, 1993).

During the last 100 years, the industrialized countries have witnessed a true revolution in population health, reflected in an increase of average life expectancy at birth of about 25 years. However, the social differences in health seem not to be narrowing. The socioeconomic differences in mortality increased in Finland between 1981 and 1990 (Karjalainen & Melkas, 1993). In Sweden, a marked increase in class-related mortality inequity took place between the 1960s and the 1980s, but this trend seems to have been broken over the last decade (National Board of Health, Sweden, 1997).

The first part of the century was dominated by diseases associated with poverty, such as infections, malnutrition, and perinatal complications. By the 1950s, cardiovascular diseases were responsible for about half of all deaths. Since 1970, cardiovascular mortality has again dropped, contributing to a recent increase in men's life expectancy.

Despite these improvements, the demand for health services is greater than ever, and most countries struggle to control their health budgets. Also, judging from the consumption of health insurance, people's health is seemingly not improving. Population studies from the Nordic countries demonstrate some increase in the reporting of symptoms, dysfunctions, and health complaints, and there is evidence for a widening socioeconomic divide in self-reported health (Whitehead, 1997). Attempts have been made to explain this "health paradox" through several mechanisms: It reflects the "medicalization" of trivial life problems; it comes from an increased dependency on medical care; it is a strategy for obtaining welfare benefits; or it reflects real increases in health problems due to psychosocial stress and other mechanisms (Barsky, 1988).

There is some evidence that life in the postindustrialized society creates health problems of a new nature. In primary health care, an increasing number of patients are complaining about vague feelings of discomfort, general pains and aches, depression and anxiety, and a number of other psychosomatic symptoms. The increased use of health insurance for sick listing, rehabilitation allowance, and disability pensions also reflects the predominance of disorders that are difficult to classify in biomedical terms.

A special problem that has been observed in Sweden and Norway over the last 10 to 15 years is an increase in chronic musculoskeletal complaints and disorders. Women are clearly more afflicted than men, especially when it comes to more generalized pains (fibromyalgia). Since 1985, a dramatic increase in disability pensioning due to such disorders has been noted in both countries, despite concurrent general improvements in the physical work environment. The double burden of women who are responsible for household duties and contribute to family income has been linked to the "new morbidity." Furthermore, a heavier psychological work demand and the introduction of new technologies such as computers have given employees new stress that some cannot handle.

Developments in Health Promotion

The Nordic countries were influential in developing the WHO Health For All by the year 2000 (HFA 2000) strategy in the late 1970s. Later, all Nordic countries issued national policy documents relating to HFA 2000 and the European regional targets (Salmela, 1991). In a governmental white paper from 1988, the overriding principles for Norway's health policy were defined as decentralization, increased primary health care, intersectoral health promotion, equity, and strengthening consumers' influence in the health services (Norwegian Ministry of Social Affairs, 1988). Later, the Norwegian parliament endorsed a policy document about health promotion in which intersectoral work at both the central and municipal levels was seen as a fundamental principle (Norwegian Ministry of Social Affairs, 1993). Priority was given to the following problem areas: psychosocial disorders, musculoskeletal disorders, accidental injuries, asthma and allergies, and health problems related to indoor climate. The strengthening of local democracy, the vitalizing of communities and neighborhoods, and the participation of the population are regarded as core tenets of health promotion policies.

All Nordic countries implemented radical legislative reforms in the 1970s and 1980s, emphasizing the role of primary health service in health care and health promotion work. The organization of primary health care was left with either the municipalities or the counties (regions), securing access to medical care, preventive services, and home-based nursing for all in need. In 1984, the new Municipality Health Services Act in Norway gave the local health authorities primary responsibility for health promotion activities, including surveillance of the population's health, advocacy about health-related matters, and the responsibility of initiating cross-sectoral preventive measures. In Sweden, the county councils were given the same tasks beginning in 1983.

These legislative changes were part of a general policy of decentralization and democratization and also reflected the broader view of health promotion as formulated in the Ottawa Charter of 1986. Despite these reforms, prevention and health promotion still struggle in the competition with curative medical services. The combat to curb rising health care costs and to meet an ever increasing demand for specialist medical care has dominated the public debate in the 1990s. A combination of professional and public expectations and economical incentives still gives preference to preventive services with questionable effectiveness, such as routine health controls, screening procedures, and single risk factor interventions.

To stimulate the local health promotion work and to gain experience with alternative strategies, a 5-year national program for development projects in health promotion was undertaken in Norway from 1989. Each year, municipalities were invited to apply for funds to finance local health promotion projects. More than 300 individual projects were given support, covering traditional public health areas as well as new approaches to community health promotion. About one third of these projects could be characterized as innovative, either in content or method. A number of the projects were based on intersectoral collaboration and public participation; most were, however, anchored in the community health sector. The low threshold in terms of planning and accountability helped many ideas get started; however, few projects satisfied more strict criteria for evaluating effectiveness. Process evaluation identified a number of critical points for developing local health promotion initiatives: The collaborating partners needed to feel the project as their own from the very beginning; early and continued involvement of local politicians helped the project gain support and increased the chances for continued funding; projects should pay attention to sustainability long before the project period ends; enthusiastic leadership can help a project grow but can also hinder broader participation and ownership; and mobilizing community groups can succeed if there is enough flexibility to allow for real influence and participation. Observe examples of this in the following case description.

> A local health promotion project in a small rural fishing community in Western Norway was initiated by the leader of the health authority as a follow-up of a community diagnosis project (Boonstra, 1990). In each subdistrict, popular meetings were held at which the results of the community health analysis was presented and discussed. The meetings identified and prioritized local health promotion action areas, and population task force groups were elected to initiate work in the selected areas. Although a previous household survey had indicated that cardiovascular diseases were seen as the most important health problem, the selected health promotion action areas were more concerned with mental and psychosocial issues, such as loneliness, lack of social meeting places, and faulty transportation systems. Health promotion work was con- ceived of by the population as a strategy for strengthening community identity and as a means for increasing the influence of the subdistricts on municipal administration and politics. Health was clearly seen in a broader perspective than individual well-be- ing and survival; rather, the survival and growth of the local communities were defined as the overall goal for health promotion action.

In Sweden, the counties (regions) assume the responsibility for all primary and secondary health services and for health promotion. This arrangement has led to an interest in planning for health development in the regions supported by regular public health reports at the national and regional level. Several of the academic institutions have engaged themselves in practical public health work, combining epidemiological methodology and social and organizational theory with action research. Recently, the influence of the WHO Sundsvall Conference on Supportive Envi- ronments in 1991 and the United Nations Conference on Environment and Development in 1992 led local Swedish authorities to establish Healthy Community networks and encourage the formulation of politically binding local Agenda 21 documents.[1]

In Denmark, much of the developmental work in public health has been linked to the WHO Healthy Cities initiative, which is a community-based approach to health development in urban settings (Price & Tsouros, 1996). Presently involving national and international networks of more than 1000 cities, the WHO Healthy cities project is based on political commitment and the establishing of structures for local health promotion and sustainable development.

Early on, Finland organized primary health care in a community model. The pioneering North Karelia project stimulated nationwide community intervention programs for cardiovascular prevention that, seemingly, contributed to a substantial reduction in cardiovascular mortality in Finland (Puska, Toumilehto, Nissinen, et al., 1995). Due to a system of central planning and decision making, public participation in community health development was limited (Salmela, 1991); however, more recently, local health promotion has been stimulated through funding and other mechanisms.

Community Accident Prevention Programs

Accidental injuries are a major public health problem worldwide. In Norway, unintentional injuries are the leading cause of death among people under 50 years old and lead to more lost years of life than cancer (Ytterstad, 1995). Also, accidental injuries represent substantial societal costs. In Sweden, annual social expenditure for personal injuries was in 1990 estimated at 63 billion SEK, the equivalent of 4% of the GNP (Jansson, 1994). The human costs of accidental injuries in the form of suffering, grief, and disability are devastating and immeasurable. In particular, children, adolescents, and the elderly are at risk. Furthermore, there are social differences in the risk of suffering unintentional injury; children of white-collar workers have much lower mortality rates than children whose parents have traditional working-class occupations (Östberg, 1996). Among adult Swedish men, the socioeconomic differences in accidental deaths have increased during the 1980s (National Board of Health, Sweden, 1997).

Accidents cannot fully be avoided, but injury is, on the other hand, not inevitable. A wide range of educational, environmental, and legislative measures can prevent accidents and injury (World Health Organization, 1989). A strategic mix of *active* (i.e., behavior-oriented) and *passive* (i.e., environment-oriented) actions is the most effective approach. Although injury control should be undertaken on all levels, the community-based model, adapting interventions to the local cultural, social, and organizational environments and emphasizing broad community participation, has emerged as the most promising model for injury prevention, although so far relatively few studies on effectiveness have been internationally published (Towner, 1994). This is rather surprising, given the importance of the problem and the fact that it is possible to detect the effects of a successful program soon after its implementation.

In both Norway and Sweden, several community-based accident prevention studies have been undertaken over the last 20 years, allowing for some accumulation of experiences and results (Table 10.1). An early study in Northern Norway demonstrated a considerable reduction in the incidence of accidental injuries in a fishing community after 2 years of systematic educational and environmental input from the local health service working in close collaboration with other public sectors and private organizations (Tellnes, 1985). Later, several quasi-experimental studies of community intervention programs confirmed that significant reductions in accidental injury rates are possible within a short time span.

In a pioneering study, Schelp (1988) developed a municipal intervention model for accident prevention using broad cooperation between local authorities, organizations, associations, and individuals. This program combined an initial organization-oriented perspective with an increasing

TABLE 10.1 Reductions in Accidental Injury Incidence After Prevention Programs

Project/ (Reference)	Study Design	Targets for Intervention	Duration (in years)	Reduction
Værøy (Tellnes, 1985)	Pre and post	All accidental injuries	2	29%
Falköping (Schelp, 1987b)	Quasi-experimental	Home accidents	3	27%
		Occupational accidents	3	28%
		Traffic accidents	3	28%
Harstad (Ytterstad, 1995)	Quasi-experimental	Burns in children	7	53%
		Traffic injuries	5	27%
		Fall fractures in the elderly	5	26%
		Skiing injuries	3	15%

citizen-oriented perspective, thus combining top-down with bottom-up strategies in a consensus-building model. The program was developed in eight steps: (a) epidemiological mapping, (b) selection of risk groups and environments, (c) forming multidisciplinary working and reference groups, (d) joint planning of the action program, (e) implementation, (f) evaluation, (g) modification, and (h) transfer of experience to the rest of the county. The preventive program consisted of (a) information and advice through local media, child health centers, and other public locations; (b) education and instruction for groups who had contact with the target groups (children, elderly, and selected occupational groups); (c) supervision through checklists and safety visits; and (d) environmental changes.

Over a 3-year period, this comprehensive program was developed and implemented in Falköping, a typical rural and semiurban municipality in the central part of Sweden. A similar municipality, Linköping, served as a comparison area. The occurrence of injuries was monitored in both municipalities through a registration system in primary health care and hospitals before and after the program. No significant changes in accidental injury incidence were noted in the comparison area. In contrast, significant reductions were observed in Falköping for all chosen targets: home accidents, occupational accidents and traffic accidents (Schelp, 1987b). In addition, a substantial fall in hospitalization days due to external violence and poisoning was noted in Falköping. After the discontinuation of the accident prevention program at the end of 1982, the outpatient injury rate leveled off and the admission rates to hospitals increased (Svanström, Schelp, et al., 1996). In 1991, the local authorities in Falköping again established a cross-sectoral organization and revitalized the program.

As Linköping had served as a comparison area, it was decided to organize a health program there, targeting (among other areas) unintentional injuries (Svanström, Ekman, Schelp, & Lindström, 1995). The experiences from Falköping were used. An intersectoral reference group for injury prevention work was formed, with representatives from the health services, municipal management, local authorities, and a variety of local organizations. In addition, a working party for the prevention of childhood injuries was set up. Special surveillance of school injuries and traffic injuries formed a basis for the intervention activities, focusing on the increased use of safety equipment, such as bicycle helmets and infant car seats, and the development of safe environments, such as playgrounds, bicycle lanes, and gym floors. Extensive information was provided to parents, households, child health care staff, and day-care staff. Over the 8 years of intervention, an average annual decrease in the incidence of hospitalized injuries in those under 14 years old was found to be 2.4% for boys and 2.1% for girls. In comparison, four "border" municipalities had an average increase of 0.6% for boys and 2.2% for girls in the same period.

In Harstad, a medium-sized town in Northern Norway, a communitywide accident prevention program was organized on the initiative of a surgeon at the local hospital (Ytterstad, 1995). Based on an established surveillance system for hospital-treated (both in- and outpatient) accidental injuries, the injury incidence rates in Harstad (population 22,000) could be compared with those of the city of Trondheim (population 134,000). In 1985, an injury prevention group (IPG) was formed in Harstad with representatives from the local hospital, the community health services, the local consumer office, police, and private and public organizations in the municipality. This group reviewed the local accident data, decided on targets for accident prevention work, and initiated interventions. The community awareness of injuries as a problem was enhanced by disseminating information from the local injury registration system to the public, including anonymous case descriptions. Also, the registry data were extensively used in rapid feedback to collaborating partners, increasing the feeling of "ownership" toward the community injury problem. The local media played an important role in the information dissemination process, in addition to direct mail and the organizational network.

The following targets were chosen for intervention in successive order by the IPG: (a) child accidents in general and burns in small children in particular, (b) traffic accidents, (c) fall fractures in the elderly, and (d) downhill skiing injuries. For all the specified targets, substantial reductions in accidental injury incidence rates were observed after intervention, ranging from 53% reduction in burns in children less than 5 years old to 15% reduction in downhill ski injuries (Table 10.1). In the comparison area, an increase in traffic injuries and fall fractures among the elderly and no change in child burns was seen during the same period.

LESSONS TO BE LEARNED

A common denominator in these community injury prevention projects has been an emphasis on creating broad intersectoral participation in public and private organizations and groups. To ensure this, a coordinating body involving the local community network was found to be essential (Schelp, 1987a; Ytterstad, 1995). The primary tasks for such a committee were to share information, analyze the situation, develop priorities, choose targets and strategies, clarify the expected performance and input from the collaborating parties, monitor progress, and make the necessary adjustments.

The projects were established as a collaborative venture among a number of public and private organizations. None of the projects were initiated by lay-group pressure alone. The most typical has been an initiative from some public health body or person, often with support from an academic institution finding an opportunity for research. In some of the later projects, the initiative has come from local political bodies.

In line with the general philosophy in community work, the projects were developed through an open-ended, transparent, cyclical process allowing for participant and population influence, democratic decisions, and accountability. A close collaboration with the local press opened up communication with citizens and more informal groups. In general, these projects were low-cost programs allowing only for a small technical secretariat and a few employed project workers. As much input as possible was directed through existing resources and services in the hope that such changes would be more sustainable after the ending of the formal project period. The hope was that more and more of the program activities would be overtaken by the public services as part of their routines. However, the experience was that over time, a certain attrition in safety concern and activities is likely to occur. Svanström, Schelp, et al. (1996) found that despite continuation of a number of individual preventive activities within each public sector, the disbanding of the Project Reference Group led to less intensive and effective work. The invisible nature of the results is one explanation for this. Another is the belief that safety work can be done once and for all. Experiences from Falköping and Harstad show, however, that continuation by some coordinating body is necessary to secure durable and expanding effects.

According to Bjärås (1991), leadership is the single most crucial factor in the maintenance of a preventive program. Some form of rooting in local institutions is required to establish and maintain a program (Ekman, 1996). Furthermore, to initiate intersectoral collaboration, committed individuals must form an "inner circle" and be advocates within their respective organizations for the program. To ensure sustained intersectoral work, a more institutionalized partnership is needed, involving the sector leadership. Also, political participation is very helpful in both establishing the program and securing the continuation of activities.

All programs relied on local injury data. Ytterstad (1995) says, "Local data (is) the locomotive of the injury prevention train" (p. 74). National statistics are of limited value for analyzing which factors contribute to the injury process (Schelp, 1987b); more important is the motivating effect of local data for preventive action and the necessity of such data for evaluation and rapid feedback. In the absence of routine registration, it is necessary to set up special surveillance systems that are both costly and difficult to run on sufficient quality. Thus, several of the experimental studies have had problems with missing data, especially in the comparison areas where no intervention team was present to keep the registration up to standards. However, based on the accumulated experiences, less costly and cumbersome surveillance systems have been developed that can more easily be fit into routine activities in primary and secondary health care (Nordic Medico-Statistical Committee, 1990).

SAFE COMMUNITIES

Based on research and the developmental work in Falköping and other early community prevention projects, a Safe Community model for injury prevention has been developed by WHO (World Health Organization, 1989). Within this concept, the municipality undertakes an injury prevention program with the following characteristics:

1. Establishment of a coordinating cross-sectoral group
2. Involvement of the local community network
3. Injury prevention that is adapted to a major population strategy involving all age-groups and environments

4. The identification of high-risk and especially vulnerable groups
5. Availability of a surveillance system
6. A sustainable preventive program
7. A process and summative evaluation
8. The identification of cooperative partners by structured organizational analysis
9. Involvement of the health services in surveillance and action programs
10. Involvement of all levels of the community
11. Dissemination of the experience through publications and other means

The idea of *safe community* is rapidly catching on among Nordic municipalities as a program for improving safety and health and thereby the quality of life for the population. The symbolic attractiveness of being recognized as a WHO Safe Community has obviously been a strong motivating factor for some politicians and decision makers. By the end of 1997, 21 municipalities were officially designated as WHO Safe Communities, forming an international network together with WHO Collaborating Centers on Injury Control.

Among the Nordic countries, Sweden has been the leader in policy and strategy formulation for injury prevention work. A national strategy document from 1991 formulated a number of intermediate and process-oriented goals, such as the dissemination of the Safe Community model and the use of standardized local injury surveillance systems. During the period 1982 through 1995, a 25% reduction in accidental deaths was observed for Sweden as a whole (National Board of Health, Sweden, 1997).

Experience says that safety planning and monitoring should be fully integrated in the managerial philosophy to be sustainable within an organization. In the Nordic countries, quality assurance and quality control are now being introduced as an integral part of management in both the private and public sectors. Very positive experiences with systematic security management schemes in the high-risk North Sea oil exploration industry have been transferred to land-based industries and even to public services. These systems require that every organization establish security standards and surveillance systems, integrate security in the planning processes, develop a security-conscious culture within the organization, and include participation from all those employed in the security work. Thus, accident prevention is seen less as an individual responsibility and more as an organizational task.

Challenges for Health Promotion in a Late-Modern Society

PUBLIC OR PRIVATE?

A central tenet in the current health promotion ideology is the active participation of the population in the planning and implementation of action. Health promotion is often conceptualized as a social movement, a channel through which individuals and groups can mobilize to change oppressive or unfavorable social conditions (Labonte, 1994). Community empowerment implies community dialogue and participation in decision making around problem definition and solutions (Wallerstein & Bernstein, 1994).

The development of the "welfare municipality" in the Nordic countries has shifted responsibility for common action from the local informal networks and neighborhoods to governmental bodies. The old tradition of *dugnad* in rural Norway, meaning unpaid work for a common purpose, has gradually been replaced by taxation-financed public services. Occasionally, members of voluntary organizations still offer their work power for a common project, such as building a church or a sports ground; however, the tendency is to see such projects as a governmental responsibility.

The voluntary organizations played an important role in developing public health services and local health care in the Nordic countries. Many preventive and curative health measures were pioneered by these organizations, such as the establishment of hospitals, maternity clinics, mother and child health centers, public health nursing, and home care for the elderly. Gradually, these functions have been overtaken by the government. Also, the pioneering work in health education and disease prevention by nongovernmental organizations has to a large extent been replaced by publicly financed activities.

In an effort to strengthen the NGOs' role, a national Coordinating Board of Health Education and Promotion was set up in Norway in the 1980s. Health promotion councils were established in each county and in many municipalities. Experience has been, however, that these bodies have problems in being recognized as partners in health promotion work by the governmental agencies.

THE CHANGING CONCEPT OF "COMMUNITY"

Health promotion has been criticized for operating with models of communities that are too simplistic; the community is seen only as a naturally bounded consensus social unit (Nilsen, 1996). Subcultural social norms, values, and hierarchies have not sufficiently been addressed in previous health promotion research, despite the ideological ambitions of the health promotion movement. The preconceived goals of health promotion initiators have largely determined the course of action. Participation by the population has assumed adherence to the program's aims and directions, with less influence on priorities and choice of action areas (Nilsen & Kraft, 1997).

When community health promotion is organized as an open-ended process, allowing for dialogue and democratic control by the citizens, local identities will influence program content and choice of action (Nilsen, 1996). Experience from several population-governed projects in Norway shows that people conceive of "health" as a broad social construct reflecting well-being, feelings of security and stability, and mutual responsibility and participation. When given the option to choose freely, people often prefer to work on issues related to social interaction and collaboration or to engage in practical projects, such as building or restoring a public house or space. Such broad psychosocial engagement is clearly in line with the ideology of modern health promotion, but population control may lead to less emphasis on other important individual or societal health determinants.

HEALTH CARE: FRIEND OR FOE?

The community health service has an ambiguous role in facilitating health promotion at the local level. Some view community health promotion as a lay alternative for health development and shun the participation of experts and authorities. Others acknowledge the leadership role of community health care in advocating for broad partnerships in health.

In the Nordic countries, primary health care is largely publicly funded and organized, either at the municipal or county level. The community health service has the double role of offering curative and preventive services to the population and promoting population health through systematic action and collaboration. The "new public health," defined as an interdisciplinary pursuit using collaborative strategies and building on public participation, can act as a strong force for community health promotion. Experiences in injury prevention testify to the leading role health professionals may take in establishing community health promotion programs. However, such leadership may also hinder broader participation unless enough sensitivity is given to the role of professionals in health promotion (Labonte, 1994).

FROM PROJECTS TO POLITICS

The ultimate goal of health promotion programs is to establish sustainable structures and functions for health. Demonstration projects are necessary to learn about implementation, processes, and outcomes but are by definition time-limited inputs with limited ability to affect population health. Developing healthy public policies has a much higher potential to achieve durable health gains. However, politicians and decision makers need to be guided to make the best investments in health. To obtain a sound scientific basis for such judgments, we still need the evidence that derives from carefully planned and conducted scientific studies. The accumulated experience in accidental injury prevention presented in this paper serves as one example of a research-based foundation of future health promotion development.

NOTE

1. Agenda 21 is the action plan for the next century that was developed at the 1992 United Nations Conference on Environment and Development in Rio de Janeiro. An important feature of Agenda 21 is the encouragement of citizens and organizations in taking part in the formulation of local policy decisions on environment, health, and sustainable development (Local Agenda 21). More information may be found at http://www.agenda21.se

11

Health and Health Promotion in Latin America

A Social Change Perspective

ABEL ARVIZU WHITTEMORE

JANET R. BUELOW

Latin America: A Brief Overview

Latin America starts with the southern border of the United States and extends through nearly 50 countries to the southernmost tips of nations near the Falkland Islands. The width of this region extends between the Caribbean and the Pacific oceans. This vast region has great variations in climate, geography, socioeconomic conditions, and culture. The United Nations has categorized the countries of Latin America into four subregions: (a) the Caribbean, with 22 islands; (b) Central America, with Belize, Costa Rica, El Salvador, Guatemala, Honduras, Mexico, Nicaragua, and Panama; (c) Tropical South America, with Bolivia, Brazil, Colombia, Ecuador, French Guiana, Guyana, Paraguay, Peru, Surinam, and Venezuela; and (d) Temperate South America, with Argentina, Chile, Uruguay, and the Falkland Islands (Marshall, 1991).

Today, most Latin American countries have some form of civilian government with elected officials. Even with the growing discontent regarding these countries' living and economic conditions, democracy is generally pervasive throughout the continent. Constitutional reforms are under way in many countries for reforms such as greater protection of citizens' rights and regional autonomy through decentralization (Pan American Health Organization [PAHO], 1995). Latin American governments generally have large military expenditures, severe foreign debt repayments, and tremendous inflation (Chelala, 1990). Most Latin American countries have enjoyed better conditions in the 1990s than they did in the 1980s. Overall, there was an average 2% per capita income growth in the 1990s. Also, the GDP growth in the typical Latin American country this decade ranged between 3% and 4% per year (Echeverria-Cota, 1996). Within each Latin American country, severe gaps may be found between the poor and the rich and between rural and urban populations. Incomes of the low- and middle-income groups are decreasing, and the wealthiest segments of the population are becoming more affluent (PAHO, 1995).

During the early 1980s, when unemployment reached the highest levels ever, strong migration trends to urban areas were experienced. Today, in many countries, the proportion of urban population is as high as 75%, and it is projected that 91% of the population increase in the rest of the century will take place in urban areas (PAHO, 1995). Historically, rural populations in Latin American countries have had the most difficult conditions. Today, almost half of the rural populations do not have access to clean water, and two thirds do not have services for the disposal of excreta and refuse. In mining areas of high mountainous areas such as the Andes, water poses a great risk to indigenous communities. Contamination results from the use of chemical fertilizers, pesticides, and organophosphate insecticides, as well as from the disposal of toxic or radioactive waste. The problem has grown to a point at which significant traces of chemical substances, as well as toxic levels of mercury, have been detected in surface water, food, and other basic nutrients necessary for survival, such as breast milk (PAHO, 1993).

Roemer (1991) contends that a nation's health system is the outcome not only of its history but also of its economic and political infrastructure. Economically, Latin American countries are recognized as consistently underfunding public health care because of their large military expenditures and foreign debt repayments. Hence, Latin American countries are classified as economically "transitional." Politically, Latin American countries are generally classified as "welfare oriented," which means that the government tries to collectivize financing and link it to organized health care delivery. This system of delivery ranges from environmental sanitation provisions and assuring human resources in the health field to bringing services to rural areas.

In most countries, a minimum of three tiers of health care systems exist: the official ministry of health, private practices for the rich minorities, and traditional medicine overseen by shamen and traditional healers (Trevelyan, 1992). However, two other health care structures—charity or "beneficencia" services and social security services—still exist as separate structures in some countries but have merged into the ministry of health in other countries. Hospitals are generally located only in urban centers and have responsibility for rural populations. Small health centers or posts are located in rural areas, with community health workers assigned to these posts (Roemer, 1991).

The social security system offers coverage to the sector of the public with "formal" employment. This system excludes all unemployed persons; those employed in the informal sector, where there is the largest increase in jobs; and all rural workers. The system thus contributes to the profound inequities in the health sector. The private health sector has experienced growth in several countries and is recognized as competition for the social security system. This system seems to incorporate new technology and to have modern facilities, which attract the population that can afford this level of services (PAHO, 1995). Table 11.1 includes an overview on health services expenditures and health status indicators.

TABLE 11.1 Summary of Selected Factors in Latin America

Demographics
- Annual rate of population increase in Latin America is approximately 2.5%.
- By the year 2000, the majority of the population (62%) will be adults between age 15 and 64 years old (PAHO, 1995).

Education
- Enrollment rates for primary school age children are between 80% and 100%, at the secondary level between 40% and 80%, and below 35% for the postsecondary level (PAHO, 1995).

Health Services Expenditures
- The average per capita health expenditure in Latin American countries was $162 in 1997, ranging from less than $50 (for Bolivia, Ecuador, and Haiti) to over $600 in the Bahamas.
- The average percentage of GDP spent on health in Latin American countries was 6.2% (Govindaraj, Chellaraj, & Murray, 1997).

Health Status
- Infant mortality rates have decreased in every country. Rates range from above 100 per 1,000 in Haiti and Bolivia to rates of below 20 per 1,000 in Chile (Bahr & Wehrhahn, 1993).
- In countries classified as in a "poverty model," more than 70% of all avoidable deaths occur in the under 15 age group. In countries considered under a "wealth model," more than 60% of the avoidable deaths occur among the population aged 45 to 64 (Curto de Casas, 1993).
- For infants, infectious and parasitic diseases were the greatest cause of mortality in most countries. For children 1 to 4 years old, violent deaths had the highest mortality rates, with accidents—other than those involving motor vehicles—accounting for the largest percentage of deaths for most countries. For the age group of 5 to 24 years, violent deaths continued to be the highest cause of mortality. As age increases, so does mortality from traffic accidents, suicide, and homicide increase, with marked increases in the 15 to 19 and 20 to 24 years groups (Chelala, 1990; Yunes, 1993).

BORDER HEALTH CONDITIONS

Between the United States and Mexico are 2,000 miles of international boundary line, with 3,889,578 Mexicans and 5,199,930 Americans living beside it. Also along this line are more than 1,500 assembly plants, or *maquiladoras*, employing over half a million individuals. The employees of these plants reside primarily in 12 bordering "sister cities" or "squatter villages," as migrants from southern areas of Mexico have responded to employment opportunities. The most populated border area is Juarez and its sister city, El Paso, which by the year 2000 is projected to have more than 2.3 million people living in the largest international metropolis in the world (Bruhn & Brandon, 1997). Border health issues have been identified as urgent problems confronting both countries.

One of the most urgent health problems identified in this area is the lack of an adequate infrastructure. The population has doubled in 11 years, but the infrastructure has not grown accordingly. It appears that neither the companies nor the governments supported more services as they built plants and encouraged towns' expansions for their employees (Moure-Eraso, Wilcox, Punnett, Copeland, & Levenstein, 1994). Aside from environmental health problems, evidence is mounting that work in maquiladora industries can be hazardous to one's health. Mexican workers employed by U.S. companies in Mexico are not protected by the OSHA standards enforced in the United States. Because more than 60% of maquiladora workers are young women, the effect of work on the reproductive health of women and potential fetuses is important. Studies have found that infants from female maquiladora workers have significantly lower birth weights when compared with international standards or comparable infant birth weights of Mexican women (Bruhn & Brandon, 1997; Eskenazi, Guendelman, & Elkin, 1993).

HEALTH PROMOTION STRUCTURES

Formal health promotion structures in Latin America can be found in programs supported by the Pan American Health Organization (PAHO), ministries of health (Bahr & Wehrhahn, 1993), state regulations (Fuenzalida-Puelma, Linares Parada, & La Vertu, 1992), nongovernmental organizations (NGOs), and universities. Reviewed here are examples of structures and premises of health promotion programs supported by some of these entities.

The Pan American Health Organization

At the First International Conference on Health Promotion in 1986, the Ottawa Charter for Health Promotion (World Health Organization, 1986) declared health promotion as "the process of enabling people to increase control over, and to improve, their health" (p. iii). Four years later, at a PAHO conference, the description of health promotion was expanded from individual efforts to community efforts involving health and social fields. Health promotion was described as "the sum activity of the population, the health services, the health authorities, and other productive and social services, aimed at improving the status of individual and collective health" (PAHO, 1991, p. 31). In 1992, at the International Conference on Health Promotion, health promotion continued to be viewed as both an individual and community effort, but the foundation for successful health promotion was expounded in the Declaration of Santafé de Bogotá (PAHO, 1992). It declared the following assumptions as a foundation of health promotion:

1. The problems of basic standards of living, as well as economic, environmental, and social inequalities must be faced and resolved.
2. An essential role of health promotion consists of identifying the factors that encourage inequity and proposing actions to alleviate their effects.
3. Public participation is important in modifying poor sanitary conditions and unhealthy behaviors.
4. The limiting of democratic practices and citizen participation in decision making contributes to violence, which contributes to public health problems.
5. Health promotion strategies must incorporate cultural traditions and social procedures that are integral for the development of human beings and societies.

With the above health promotion premises, the official PAHO structure for health promotion is the Division of Health Promotion and Protection. Within this division, the priority areas are (a) healthy development of adolescents, with emphases on healthy and safe sexual practices, to address problems such as HIV/AIDS and adolescent pregnancies, drug addiction, tobacco and alcohol consumption, violence, accidents, and injuries; (b) promotion of healthy cities or communities at the local level, while strengthening the decentralization process and the role of citizens; and (c) policies addressing problems associated with poverty, demographic changes, rapid urbanization, and industrialization. Some associated problems include the growth of criminal activities, rising rates of violence and impairments caused by violence, and the rising incidence of noncommunicable diseases associated with unhealthy habits and behaviors and their subsequent impairments (PAHO, 1995).

The Division of Health Promotion and Protection has several technical programs and centers that draw upon official documents and individual country ministries of health for facilitating health promotion activities. The technical programs within this division are the Healthy Lifestyles and Mental Health Program, a family health and population program that includes an adolescent health program, and a food and nutrition program. The centers within the division of Health Promotion and Protection are the Institute of Nutrition of Central America and Panama (INCAP), Caribbean Food and Nutrition Institute (CFNI), and Latin American Center for Perinatology and Human Development (CLAP).

Ideally, all of the programs facilitated through the Division are to give priority to the social, cultural, and political factors that influence the maintenance, improvement, and restoration of health and well-being. Examples of some of their programs include research and intervention programs geared to achieve nonviolent societies, training seminars and courses for adolescent health professionals, food security activities, and programs to combat malnutrition problems such as protein, vitamin A, and iron deficiencies.

Within PAHO, the fundamental primary commitment of health promotion advocates is the recognition that health is conditioned by political, economic, social, cultural, environmental, and biological factors and that health promotion is a strategy to change these conditioning factors. In other words, health promotion includes acting as an agent of change in society (PAHO, 1995).

University Programs

A survey of all universities in Central and South America identified many health promotion programs in progress for nutrition and fitness programs (Lara-Pantin, 1993). These programs, although quite progressive for their targeted populations, appear to be very individualistic and are not coordinated with other programs within their country.

Several countries had universities involved in programs related to their geographic, occupational, or socioeconomic conditions. In Brazil, the Center of Study for Physical Fitness–Research Laboratory defined physical fitness parameters for the Brazilian population 7 through 18 years old and identified differences according to socioeconomic status. Another program in Brazil involved professors investigating nutritional status, metabolic changes, and adaptation to different types of physical activities. In Peru, the Department of Nutrition of the German-Peruvian Agreement for Andean Cultures (COPACA) studied nutrition and physical fitness in relation to work performance and geographical conditions in the area.

Several other countries reported on programs for their elite athletes. In Chile, the Department of Food Sciences and Technology worked on the development of nutritional products for athletes using locally available food sources and technology. In Mexico, the National Institute of Nutrition participates in activities addressed to athletes for various health disciplines. In Columbia, schools of dietetics included in their curricula a course on nutrition and fitness followed by dietetic students involved with evaluating the nutritional status of athletes. Also, the federal agency for sports, Coldeportes, created a foundation to help elite athletes needing economical support for their careers with medical, nutritional, social, and psychological assistance.

Issues Affecting Health Promotion

Most health beliefs and practices are derived from a rich array of ethnic and historical traditions. These traditions also influence health promotion behaviors found within a community. Latin American countries have some unique cultural beliefs that must be considered when designing effective health promotion programs. In particular, the cultural roots of the population, perceptions of health and illness, and utilization practices of traditional health providers must be considered for their impact on health promotion behaviors.

CULTURAL ROOTS

Ten percent of the Latin American population is composed of indigenous people. Among all the Americas, there are approximately 42 million indigenous peoples, distributed among 400 ethnic groups. This population can be divided into four groups (PAHO, 1993).

The first group has approximately 18 million and includes the indigenous peoples of Meso-America, mainly the Maya of Mexico and Guatemala, followed in decreasing order by other ethnic groups living in Mexico, Belize, Honduras, El Salvador, Panama, Nicaragua, and Costa Rica. The second group, estimated at around 20 million, is made up principally of Quechua and Aymara, who are concentrated today in the Andean countries, mainly Bolivia, Peru, and Ecuador and, to a lesser degree, Venezuela, Colombia, and Chile. These two groups make up more than 80% of the indigenous population of the Americas.

The third group has approximately 3 million people and includes a heterogeneous conglomerate of Indian groups and nations who live in the subarctic regions and in various settlements in Canada and the United States. Also, some live in the Caribbean islands, Venezuela, Brazil, Paraguay, Argentina, and Chile. The last group is an indigenous population of seasonal migrants. They generally follow the harvests, and some have become permanent migrants in medium-sized and large cities of Latin America and the United States.

Most Latin American countries have little or no information on the health status of their indigenous populations, as information in the disease registries is not separated by ethnic group. However, information available from secondary sources provides evidence that the levels of health of these populations are several times below the national averages.

Diseases that characterize indigenous peoples of the Latin American region are similar to those that plague other socioeconomically disadvantaged groups. Viral diseases (influenza, measles, dengue, poliomyelitis, viral respiratory diseases, hepatitis B, etc.) frequently explode into epidemics. The prevalence of diseases endemic to tropical and subtropical areas (e.g., leishmaniasis and onchocerciasis) remains high and especially affects those human settlements where indigenous people are a majority. Other communicable diseases such as tuberculosis and malaria are on the rise, and there are high incidence rates and lethality of cholera. Mental disorders and problems are also growing. Stress-related disorders, including violence toward others, depression, and suicide, as well as accidental and violent death, joint abuse of alcohol, tobacco, and other substances are problems that show an increasingly high prevalence among young and adult indigenous people of both sexes. Malnutrition problems include protein-calorie malnutrition and deficiencies in micronutrients, especially iron, vitamin A, and iodine.

It is recognized that the current health situation of the indigenous peoples is the result of a historical process that fostered dependency, loss of identity, and marginalization. The indigenous peoples have a shorter life expectancy than homologous national groups, higher mortality, and a distinct and changing morbidity profile that reflects a lower standard of living, social status, and level of acculturation, as well as a higher risk of disease and death (PAHO, 1993).

PERCEPTIONS OF HEALTH AND ILLNESS

Perceptions of health and illness are influenced by many factors and circumstances within Latin America. However, similarities have been found in definitions of health and illness, as well in actions taken to maintain health and control illness. Health promoting behaviors, in turn, are influenced by these health perception factors and modified by demographic factors and personal circumstances.

Descriptions of good health provided by Mexicans in a study by Adams-McDarty (1996) includes being physically fit, having no persistent pain and discomfort, being happy or content, and being able to work and maintain a high level of physical activity. Other descriptions of health include having a "joy of life" and "harmony with nature." Illness was described as improper functioning of the body, inability to work, physiological symptoms, psychological illness, and sadness.

When asked about health maintenance activities, diet and exercise actions were most frequently mentioned. Examples of dietary practices included eating a variety of foods; limiting meat and fat intake; not eating too much; careful purchasing, cleaning, and cooking of foods; and boiling water. When asked about illness actions, responses included going to the doctor, drinking herbal teas, resting, taking medicine, and drinking liquids.

Using the Health-Promoting Lifestyle Profile to measure the frequency of health promoting behaviors, both Kuster and Fong (1993) and Walker, Kerr, Pender, and Sechrist (1990) found similarities between Latin Americans and their northern counterparts. The highest area of health promotion was self-actualization, with the other areas following, respectively: interpersonal support, nutrition, stress management, health responsibility, and exercise. Also, as with North Americans, age, education, and income correlated significantly and positively with scores. Significant differences were found between males and females, with males reporting more exercise than females. Also, married or partnered people scored significantly higher with nutrition than single people but lower on exercise.

FOLK MEDICINE

A form of folk medicine based on the humoral medicine of Western Europe was brought to the Americas by the conquistadors. The conquistadors then mixed their views of health and sickness with those of the American natives. Central tenets now recognized in Latin American folk medicine are, first, the social or kin network is very important in diagnosing and treating illness; second, the relationship between religion and illness is significant; and third, there appears to be great consistency of beliefs among communities about symptoms, etiology, and regimens of healing (Krajewski-Jaime, 1991).

Pachter (1994) studied individuals who used both folk healers and Western biomedicine in parallel. He found that people often go to biomedical practitioners for relief of symptoms and, simultaneously, use a folk therapist to eliminate the cause of the illness. Also, many go to folk therapists due to easier access, economic constraints, linguistic considerations, and uncertainty regarding the actual diagnosis. One reason identified as to why traditional folk healing may be used was that modern medicine cannot eliminate chronic problems and declining health in old age. Other reasons included the impersonal and disrespectful treatments by formal health care providers and fears that physicians actually do more harm than good. Overall, however, economic hardships were the most important factors inhibiting the use of biomedical practitioners.

Several organizations have developed programs to encourage an understanding of traditional folk healing. These programs are generally of two types: (a) efforts to preserve traditional medicines and (b) programs to help health practitioners become more sensitive and effective with a nation's population (Trevelyan, 1992).

One United Kingdom charity, Health Unlimited, tries to develop a position of respect for shamanistic practices. They help rebuild the status of these practices by working with traditional healers in their communities. They are also making a collection of traditionally used plant cures and spreading this information among the communities (Trevelyan, 1992). Another program in Mexico is conducted from an academic hospital. With this program, weekly meetings are held with medical students, anthropologists, and historians regarding traditional Mexican medical systems. These meetings are meant to stimulate practicing physicians to have a more humanistic approach in the care of their patients. In this program, students experience contact with patients in public hospitals and then become *pasantes* in small villages (Vargas & Casillas, 1989).

In Nicaragua, a program with similar goals is the Nicaragua Health Fund. This project aims to integrate traditional medicine into the current health system. This is done through a training program promoting traditional medicine use among *brigadistas* (voluntary health workers), midwives, nurses, doctors, and students. Additionally, a farm was set up with 22 medicinal plants grown for use in this program (Trevelyan, 1992).

Latin American countries together established the TAMILLE network in 1984 as an interregional scientific network that seeks a better understanding of traditional medicine. It produced a handbook listing about 300 plants and their elements and uses. Similarly, in Honduras, a nongovernmental movement called EDUCSA sponsors a program that aims to undertake research into medicinal plants to identify, register, and classify them in the indigenous communities. It may also set up traditional medicine centers that serve the purposes of treating and preventing diseases, as well as documenting the healer's special knowledge (Trevelyan, 1992).

International Organizations and Health Promotion Programs

Although the World Health Organization (WHO) is recognized as the largest international health care organization, the Pan American Health Organization (PAHO), the World Bank, and development assistance organizations also play a significant role in the promotion of health in Latin America (Basch, 1991).

THE PAN AMERICAN HEALTH ORGANIZATION

PAHO is one of six specialized organizations of the Organization of American States and is linked to the United Nations through the World Health Organization Regional Office for the Americas. A portion of the PAHO budget comes from WHO and the United Nations. Thirty-five countries of the Americas are members, as well as France, the United Kingdom, and the Netherlands, all of whom have "participating" status. The aim of PAHO is to promote and coordinate efforts to combat disease, lengthen life, and promote physical and mental health. PAHO has six zones, with headquarters in Washington, DC, Mexico City, Guatemala City, Caracas, Lima, and Rio de Janeiro. Its major work consists of cooperating with member governments to improve public health services, furnishing consultants for technical problems, organizing seminars and training courses, and collecting and distributing epidemiologic and vital health statistics (Basch, 1991).

THE WORLD BANK

The World Bank primarily focuses on supporting national and regional economic reform efforts, financial sector restructuring, and human development through both financial and technical assistance, but it has adopted a formal policy regarding awareness of the health consequences of its projects and efforts to minimize adverse effects on health resulting from its lending for industrial development (Basch, 1991). Since 1980, the bank has supported some specific health-related projects such as the development of basic health infrastructures, training of community health workers, promotion of nutrition, and prevention and control of endemic and epidemic diseases. Also, the World Bank is helping governments redefine their role in the health sector. While there are five major institutional changes being recommended (Bossert, Hsiao, Barrera, Alarcon, Leo, & Casares, 1998), in general the World Bank is encouraging governments to diminish the role of providing direct services while creating a "friendly environment" for nongovernmental involvement and increased competition among service providers (Echeverria-Cota, 1996). This is particularly evident in the World Bank's new health policy of "Investing in Health" where health is defined as a private responsibility and health care as a private good (Laurell & Arellano, 1996), and whose methodological approach has not escaped critical review (Paalman, Bekedam, Hawken, & Nyheim, 1998).

DEVELOPMENT ASSISTANCE ORGANIZATIONS

After World War II, international politico-economic alliances became prominent and national agencies were created for official "development assistance." The United States provides international assistance primarily through the Department of State and the Agency for International Development (AID). However, government assistance at a smaller level is also provided through international divisions of the National Institutes of Health, the Social Security Administration, and the Department of Defense. Donor countries with similar interests and development assistance agencies include Japan, the Scandinavian nations, Canada, the Netherlands, Great Britain, Australia, and Germany (Basch, 1991).

Thousands of private voluntary organizations or nongovernmental organizations (NGOs) based in industrialized countries provide services and funding for Latin American nations. Some of these agencies receive substantial funding from their governments and others obtain private contributions only. Many of these organizations are religiously sponsored and are centralized within denominations such as the Mennonite Central Committee, Lutheran World Relief, and Catholic Relief Services of the Roman Catholic Church. Other organizations are private, nonde-nominational foundations with a mission for international health work. One of the most recognized and largest foundations in international health is the Rockefeller Foundation, which, in its 38 years of operation, has cooperated with 75 governments in campaigns for 21 separate diseases or health problems, including its successful campaign in Brazil against the African mosquito, *Anopheles gambiae*. In addition, the foundation has built and operated field laboratories in many countries, training local scientists in methods of investigating and combating endemic diseases.

Health Promotion in Latin America

A MODEL AND EXAMPLES DEPICTING INTERVENTION STRATEGIES

A comprehensive review of the research-based literature of health promotion programs in Latin American covering the 8-year period from 1990 through 1997 reveals that these programs differ according to type, unit of focus, and the extent of the health behavior change being sought. With respect to the first component, current health promotion programs in Latin America cover the broad spectrum of community health: maternal-child health, child health, chemical health, environmental health, mental health, sexual health, and women's health. The latter two components (unit of focus and degree of change) are very similar to the dimensions found in Wilson's typology of social change (Wilson, 1973). As health promotion has as its aim the goal of social change, it seems appropriate to use Wilson's model (Table 11.2) to present some of the highlights of contemporary health promotion efforts in Latin America.

According to Harper (1989), social change efforts can be distinguished along two dimensions. First is the unit of focus: Is the change effort being directed to changing the character of individuals and their behavior (expressive change) or are the change interventions an attempt to change the structure of society (instrumental change)? Second is the degree of change, with *reform* efforts seeking to bring about modest changes within an existing system (individual or societal) and *radical* change aiming toward fundamental changes in the system (individual or societal). Using these two sets of dimensions can lead to a four-cell matrix reflecting Wilson's typology, consisting of (a) alternative change, which involves interventions seeking to bring about partial change in individuals, (b) redemptive change, which entails interventions aiming to bring about total change in individuals, (c) reformative change, in which interventions attempt to bring about partial change in supraindividual systems, and (d) transformative change, whose successful attempts result in total change in social structures.

The ensuing discussion will focus on each of these cells (Table 11.2) from a health promotion perspective: first, by presenting a health-compatible theory that is representative of the cell and, second, by highlighting some contemporary health promotion programs that depict the particular change intervention corresponding to the cell.

is, to a large extent, collectively shared and socially normed" (p. 414). Such egalitarian expectations in maternal-child health can potentially lead to the grounding of other areas of health promotion efforts on both biomedical and indigenous systems.

Such empowering social and health efforts are also evident in women's programs for which Freire's theory serves as the basic foundation. With increased health hazards such as AIDS (Plata, 1992), as well as cultural expectations influencing the use of contraceptives, family size, appropriateness of breast-feeding, and gender roles, women's biological, psychological, social, and political life experiences are significantly affected. One Mexican program recognizing that women's health entails more than a disease orientation is a health education program for female university workers from cleaning and cafeteria work units (Cardaci, 1994). This program acknowledges a need for a gender-based analysis of women's health that calls for a reconfiguration of women's social and institutional lives.

Likewise, with the increased concern over sexual experience at younger ages and the absence of contraception among young adults in Latin America (Morris, 1992), empowering health promotion programs have been developed for gay men. But again, consistent with Freire's theory, not only did the approach of an HIV/AIDS prevention program in Mexico call for empowerment outcomes, but the intervention itself also consisted of an empowering process (Zimmerman, Ramirez-Valles, Suarez, de la Rosa, & Castro, 1997). The results suggest not only increased HIV/AIDS knowledge and preventive behavior, but also an "intervention that generated community change initiated by participants" (Zimmerman, 1997, p. 177).

"Blended" Health Promotion Programs: Theories and Approaches

An attempt has been made in the discussion above to categorize health promotion programs in Latin America along a couple of dimensions with a corresponding theoretical framework, but programs abound that incorporate or can fall under more than one conceptual umbrella. Although not based in Latin America, one alcohol and substance abuse prevention program in New Mexico incorporated both Rogers' protection-motivation theory and Freire's social change theory. The program was geared to adolescents from high-risk communities. Its results revealed three stages of self-identity changes: action orientation of care, individual responsibility to act, and social responsibility to act.

This is consistent with an HIV/AIDS prevention program for female sexual partners of injection drug users in Mexico that used a triad of theories: Freire's social change, Bandura's social learning, and Werner's "barefoot doctor" community health care. The results of the intervention indicated behavioral changes stemming "from an increase in the degree of self-esteem, self-efficacy, and awareness of the social, economic, and political constraints of their lives" (Ferreira-Pinto & Ramos, 1995).

But regardless of whether there is one or a multitude of explicit or implicit driving theories being used, the Latin American programs described above all share a social change orientation. This orientation is not without its critics, who argue that these programs are based on a "romantic-idealistic" position that asserts that populations are already endowed with knowledge and know-how to autonomously define and organize their own health education projects, to produce their own educational materials, and even to conduct the teaching process by themselves" (Cardaci, 1997, p. 20). Furthermore, it is argued that specific or micro-health objectives and the more general objective of global social change require different means. In addition, the warning is given that "empowering people requires more than simply giving oppression a name, confronting it, or even getting into helping and educative relationships with local community workers. If uncritically embraced, empowering practices can lead to the many abuses they seek to redress, that is, the further disempowerment of people" (Cardaci, 1997, p. 22). The response—from proponents of health promotion within a social change framework—has been that, given the political and social dynamics in most of Latin America, the interaction of individual and community change processes is tightly interwoven.

This intertwined relationship between individual and community change is especially evident in settings where there are culturally prescribed means of prevention and intervention for the individual. In Garifuna communities in Belize, for example, wife-beating is virtually unknown due to women (with the help of the community) leaving abusive husbands. Intervention (on the part of the community) is inevitable due to a culturally sanctioned right and duty to intervene— particularly on the part of the women's kin (Kerns, 1992). This premise is the foundation for many recent women's health projects being implemented by various NGOs and community-based organizations (Manderson & Mark, 1997).

Perhaps a solution in "formal" health promotion interventions can be to embrace both the "romantic-idealistic" approach as well as an assistive approach. Project *Verdad*, a community development approach to health in Mexico, began by acknowledging Rothman's (1979) three possible models of community organization: (a) locality development, in which "the community is empowered to solve problems on its own"; (b) social planning, in which "experts enter a community, diagnose the problem, and then propose a solution"; and (c) social action, in which "an outsider acts as an advocate to clarify social issues and lead the community in an effort to change their society" (Byrd, 1992, p. 16). However, in the words of the project staff:

> We often found that communities were unable to see how serious some health problems might be. The compromise was to insist on the maximum amount of community involvement, but to "push" certain issues that were clearly important to the health of the residents. . . . This seemed to be the best possible blend of locality development and social planning. (Byrd, 1992, p. 20)

This compromise, however, does not elude the concerns of some that

> the reputed benefits of community participation . . . are just that—reputed. . . . Coupled with the additional challenges posed by the meaning of participation, community participation is a far more complicated idea and initiative than it appears at first, which in turn, hinders a final judgement with respect to the value of community participation overall. (Zakus & Lysack, 1998, pp. 3-4)

ISSUES IN PLANNING, INITIATING, AND IMPLEMENTING PROGRAMS

The use and balance of locality development and social planning, however, demands health professionals who are fully prepared to proceed with the planning, initiating, and implementation of health promotion programs. *Proyecto Zapotlan* in Mexico, for example, functions as a field school for university students in the health professions. Complete with a curriculum that includes historical, cultural, and health promotion components, the program's primary aim is to provide "an experiential, community-wide infrastructure that offers community-based education opportunities" to the community (Toledo, 1996, p. 45). Operating on a multi-university and regional basis is the Panamerican Federation of Associations of Medical Schools' (PAFAMS) agenda for the future (Pulido, 1989). In an attempt to overcome planning, initiation, and implementation challenges faced by physicians in their health promotion efforts, PAFAMS has established a database of information on medical education, developed a program to integrate medical education and health care services within individual communities, and developed a leadership program to nurture individuals who will be instrumental in developing community-based health services. In recent years, the Kellogg Foundation has extended its support for similar initiatives throughout Latin America, in an attempt to link universities with a community and its health system (Kisil & Chaves, 1994).

Other health professionals, however, can also play a significant role in the promotion of health in a community. Nurses who have been armed with cultural sensitivity and knowledge should be ideally suited to provide holistic health care (Castiglia, 1994; Quinn, 1997). And, increasingly, health professionals such as pharmacists are being viewed as essential to community-based health education. This is especially true in such areas as the prevention and treatment of sexually transmitted diseases (Pick et al., 1996). Whatever the health profession, however, it should be clear that the greatest impact on health professionals and a community will occur not in the hospital setting but outside it, as Ryan, Martinez, and Pelto (1996) make clear.

There are some additional elements to consider besides experience in a community setting and cultural awareness, along with an ability to re-form the boundaries of one's profession with respect to health promotion. These elements include the acquisition of specific knowledge and skills that are essential to the efficiency and effectiveness of health promotion efforts in Latin America. Briefly, the specific knowledge and skills needed correspond to

1. community health-appropriate management tools (Puentes-Markides & Garrett, 1996; Ramiro Montealegre, 1991) that are culture-specific (Hofstede, 1993),
2. health education methodologies (Rice & Valdivia, 1991), and
3. evaluation and research (Belizan et al., 1995).

The practical dimensions of the first two are readily apparent, but there must be equal recognition of the value of enabling practitioners to evaluate interventions. As Belizan and colleagues (1995) noted in connection to their health education program for pregnant women,

> Health education is claimed as a major component of health activities. However, there is little firm evidence about its effect and about how to enhance its effectiveness. . . . The results shown in this study are another evidence of interventions where the rationale looks appropriate, but the evaluation failed to demonstrate any benefit. . . . Health workers, particularly those in developing countries where resources are poor, must implement actions only when those actions have demonstrated significant benefits. (pp. 898-899)

There is encouraging evidence of an increased appreciation among public health professionals in Latin America to function as scholar-practitioners (Pellegrini, Goldbaum, & Silvi, 1997).

In short, the key issue pertaining to the successful planning, initiating, and implementing of health promotion programs lies with the education and training of change agents—health professionals themselves. It should be noted, however, that this is an issue that is of equal concern and applicability to developed countries. Sherraden and Wallace (1992), for example, have examined the parallel developments and challenges of community health services in Mexico and the United States.

KEY FINDINGS FROM PRACTICE AND RESEARCH IN HEALTH PROMOTION

Three key findings can be identified from this examination of health promotion programs and research. All are consistent with previous assessments (Gillies, 1998; Rice, 1988; Zakus & Lysack, 1998):

- The level of community participation in health may include the use of health services, cooperation with health services initiatives, and participation in decision making in health services. The type and level of participation will be, to a large extent, determined by the existing political structure and health care delivery system. The more effective community health programs are those that are comprehensive, community supportive, and built on existing local structures.

- Unfortunately, the prevailing attitude is still that health is the provenance of "experts," responsibility for health belongs solely to government personnel, and community health actions are the domain of designated community leaders and not the community as a whole.

- Yet, the more effective health promotion programs are those that incorporate incentives and use active methods such as theater, songs, fairs, group dynamics, self-discovery, self-care, and self-sufficiency at the community level. Those least effective involve passive health education measures and traditional curative approaches to health care.

LESSONS FOR PRACTICE, THEORY, AND OVERALL COMMUNITY DEVELOPMENT STRATEGY

We can identify two general lessons that have had and will continue to have enormous implications with respect to the practice, theory, and overall community development associated with health promotion efforts: (a) decentralization is a fact of life within major health sector reform initiatives in Latin America, and (b) there is a need for a multiparadigmatic approach to community health and healing.

Decentralization

Essentially, decentralization is the "transfer of power from central government to regions, districts, and/or provider institutions, either within the health sector or under local governments"

(Valentine, 1998, p. 6). A conceptual framework has been developed by the Pan American Health Organization (1997) to assist countries in this transition. In addition, WHO has initiated a multicountry study of decentralization and health system change (Valentine, 1998). Preliminary findings, however, as in the case study of Colombia's ministry of health, do reveal some recommendations (Bossert, Hsiao, Barrera, Alarcon, Casares, M. L., & Casares, C., 1998).

A Multiparadigmatic Approach

The persistent existence of both folk healing and conventional health care in Latin America calls for a holism in community health efforts that is based on an expansive view of the human experience. What is needed is a view that acknowledges the unity of mind, body, and spirit and that acknowledges humans as unified systems with spiritual, social, and environmental aspects that are central to healing.

Engebretson (1997) has developed a multiparadigmatic model that, although intended for the nursing discipline, has applicability to health promotion theory and practice. Engebretson's model allows for the acceptance of many complementary approaches to healing, all of which originate and operate within a cultural context. Furthermore, no single health profession, through its approaches and techniques, has a monopoly on truth with respect to health and healing. There is more than one way of knowing and healing, and folk healers have a legitimate role in healing a community. Indeed, there is a growing recognition of this within the medical profession (Dacher, 1995, 1996a, 1996b) as well as in the nursing profession (Engebretson, 1994; Quinn, 1992).

LIKELY FUTURE DIRECTIONS: BARRIERS, OPPORTUNITIES, AND SPECIAL CHALLENGES

Lessons are still being learned about the past and present, but future macrolevel prospects and challenges that will affect health promotion efforts in Latin America are already upon us (Alleyne, 1995; Puentes-Markides & Garrett, 1996; Shediac-Rizkallah & Bone, 1998):

- The distinction between the strictly national and the international will continue to grow more nebulous—particularly in such areas as environmental degradation, drug trafficking, disease, and population problems. The challenge will be to determine ways whereby a Latin American state, with very limited possibilities for acting extranationally, can influence matters that affect its security but whose origins lie outside its borders.
- There will continue to be an increasing recognition of the importance of the environment (particularly its development). The challenge is to see that more attention in environmental policy discussions is given to (a) the preservation, protection, and restoration of the environment and (b) human health and well-being. This is critical in light of those environmentally induced health problems that are on the rise.
- There appears to be no definitive reduction in the level of inequality or inequity that Latin American countries have been experiencing, and poverty continues to grow more acute. These inequities are in terms of rural and urban distribution of services, as well as gender and ethnicity. Hence, one of the major challenges in Latin America will be to continue to develop interventions to remedy these inequalities.

* The attainment of better health will be a great challenge, particularly because it will depend on the interplay of factors in many sectors. Instead of being directed toward socioeconomic development, the focus in the future should be on human development, which includes health, education, a healthy environment, and civil rights (participatory democracy and human rights).

* Ongoing epidemics of various forms—infectious diseases, noncommunicable diseases (e.g., cardiovascular), and interpersonal violence—will need to be controlled and prevented.

* Women's health issues beyond those linked solely to women's reproductive functions must be addressed.

* The health problems of the indigenous population must be addressed.

* Community participation, which is the pillar of health promotion in Latin America, is still merely a slogan. With the emerging maturity of democracy and the increasing momentum of the *municipios saludables* (healthy municipalities) decentralization movement, however, increased local expressions of citizenship rights and direct involvement in the application of health promotion strategies can be expected (Restrepo, Llanos, Contreras, Rocabado, Gross, Suarez, & Gonzalez, 1995; Wallerstein, 1998).

In closing, as we look to the future and its challenges, perhaps we would do well to remember the words of the shepherd boy Santiago: "That's what alchemists do. They show that, when we strive to become better than we are, everything around us becomes better, too" (Coelho, 1993, p. 158).

12

Emerging Public and Private Health Sector Partnerships

Selected U.S. Experiences

LEE KINGSBURY

The health care system in the United States is continuing to undergo sweeping changes. Both the private health (medical) delivery and the public health sectors are being challenged by structural changes and fiscal constraints. Examples of these changes include the formation of new corporate entities emphasizing integration of services, downsizing, managed care, and the privatization of some public health services. These factors are encouraging the development of new partnerships between public and private entities and causing a reexamination of the roles both sectors play in improving health in communities (Lasker & the Committee on Medicine and Public Health, 1997).

Although the fundamental long-term goal of both the public health and private health care sectors is to improve health, there are significant differences in how each approaches the goal. Until recently, these two sectors tended to operate quite independently of each other, almost in different spheres. When representatives of these two sectors came together, they often even viewed each other with suspicion (Coye, 1995). However, the trends in both sectors are now presenting new opportunities and generating increased interest in prevention and public health models. Despite significant challenges and historical separation, the public and private sectors are beginning to come together in new ways to improve the health of the communities they serve.

Among public health professionals there is renewed interest in partnerships which enhance the core functions or essential responsibilities of public health: (a) providing information to the community by assessing health status, health needs, disease threats, and health services—this includes surveillance and epidemiologic investigations, as well as identification of behavioral risk factors, environmental hazards, and major health determinants; (b) bringing the community together to plan for and mobilize resources to improve health; and (c) assuring the availability of quality individual, family, and public health services to the entire community, including a proactive emphasis on health protection and promotion and capacity to respond on an emergency basis to unanticipated disease and conditions and events threatening community health (Baker et al., 1994). Although these functions are receiving more attention by both state and local governmental public health agencies, the traditional public sector role of service delivery to special and indigent populations is decreasing. This role is being "reassigned" to the private sector as states contract with managed care organizations to provide health care services for their Medicaid and Medicare recipients.

The private sector has been both initiating and responding to mass restructuring, including changes in the nature of reimbursement for services. What was once a system of independently operated hospitals and clinics is now becoming a system made up of large consolidated, integrated service systems. At the same time, traditional insurance models are rapidly becoming managed care models that integrate the financing and delivery of health care services (Macro International, 1996). Driving these changes have been serious and widespread concerns of the public about the growth of health care spending, concerns of business and industry leaders about future financial obligations to provide health benefits for employees, and concerns of the health care industry related to the absorption of losses for charity care. These rapid changes and concerns, among other things, are providing new opportunities for partnerships on prevention. According to a report from the Centers for Disease Control and Prevention's Managed Care Working Group, managed care organizations (MCOs) can play a powerful role in prevention for at least three reasons: (a) They are rapidly becoming a major source of health care for those enrolled in employer-funded and publicly funded programs; (b) MCOs are developing systems to measure performance and improve the quality of services, including preventive services; (c) MCOs take responsibility for defined populations and are accountable to purchasers, individual consumers, and federal and state regulatory agencies for desired outcomes (Center for Disease Control and Prevention, 1995).

Meanwhile, our understanding of the nature of health and its determinants is also progressing. There is a wider recognition in the United States that health encompasses well-being as well as the absence of illness; that health depends not only on medical care but on other factors as well (Durch, Bailey, & Stoto, 1997). According to the 1997 Jakarta Declaration on Health Promotion in the 21st Century, prerequisites for health are peace, shelter, education, social security, social relations, food, income, empowerment of women, a stable ecosystem, sustainable resource use, social justice, respect for human rights, and equity. Above all, poverty is the greatest threat to health. This continuing expansion in our understanding of what affects health provides the basis for looking to segments of the community beyond the traditional health-focused organizations to solve health problems. It points to the need for multidisciplinary and multisector approaches. The prerequisites identified above represent a complex set of social health factors that requires solutions far beyond the resources and commitment of either the private health or public health sector. Broader community development strategies (see Chapter 1 for a discussion on Healthy Cities initiatives) must complement these emerging local partnerships.

As the understanding of the determinants of health has expanded, so has an appreciation grown of the health of a community being a shared responsibility of all its members (Durch et al., 1997). Bringing many new partners together has great potential to achieve public health goals, but creating effective relationships and defining roles among them add complexity to community

References

Abrams, D. B., Boutwell, B. B., Grizzle, J. E., Heimendinger, J., Sorensen, G., & Varnes, J. (1994). Cancer control at the workplace: The Working Well Trial. *Preventive Medicine, 23*, 15-27.

Abrams, D. B., Elder, J. P., Carleton, R. A., Lasater, T. M., & Artz, L. M. (1986). Social learning principles for organizational health promotion: An integrated approach. In M. F. Cataldo & T. J. Coates (Eds.), *Health and industry: A behavioral medicine perspective* (pp. 28-51). New York: Wiley.

Abramson, J. H., Gofin, R., Hopp, C., Gofin, J., Donchin, M., & Habib, J. (1981). Evaluation of a community program for the control of cardiovascular risk factors: The CHAD program in Jerusalem. *Israel Journal of Medical Science, 17*(2-3), 201-212.

Adams, M. J., & Hollowell, J. G. (1992). Community-based projects for the prevention of developmental disabilities. *Mental Retardation, 30*(6), 331-336.

Adams-McDarty, K. (1996). Perceptions of health and illness in Mexico. *Journal of Multicultural Nursing & Health, 2*(2), 18-22.

Administrative Committee on Coordination/Sub-Committee on Nutrition (United Nations). (1997). *Third report on the world nutrition situation.* Geneva: World Health Organization.

Airhihenbuwa, C. O. (1993). Health promotion and disease prevention strategies for African-American: A conceptual model. In R. L. Braithwaite & S. E. Taylor (Eds.), *Health issues in the Black community* (pp. 267-277). San Francisco, CA: Jossey-Bass.

Ajzen, I. (1991). The theory of planned behavior. *Organizational Behavior and Human Decision Processes, 50*, 179-211.

Ajzen, I., & Fishbein, M. (1980). *Understanding attitudes and predicting social behavior.* Englewood Cliffs, NJ: Prentice Hall.

Alcalay, R., Ghee, A., & Scrimshaw, S. (1993). Designing prenatal care messages for low-income Mexican women. *Public Health Reports, 108*(3), 354-362.

Alinsky, S. (1946). *Reveille for radicals.* Chicago, IL: University of Chicago Press.

Alleyne, G. (1995). Prospects and challenges for health in the Americas. *Bulletin of the Pan American Health Organization, 29*(3), 264-271.

Altman, D. G. (1995). Sustaining interventions in community systems: On the relationship between researchers and communities. *Health Psychology, 14*, 526-536.

Altman, D. G., Endres, J., Linzer, J., Lorig, K., Howard-Pitney, B., & Rogers, T. (1991). Obstacles to and future goals of ten comprehensive community health promotion projects. *Journal of Community Health, 16*, 299-314.

Alvarez Larrauri, S. (1994). Oral rehydration therapy promotion: An education-communication experiment. *Promotion & Education, 1*(4), 22-26, 48.

America's Children: Key National Indicators of Well Being. (1998, July.) Washington, DC: National Institute of Drug Abuse, Department of Health and Human Services, Publication 065-000-01162-0.

Amezcua, C., McAlister, A., Ramirez, A., & Espinoza, R. (1990). A Su Salud: Health promotion in a Mexican-American border community. In N. Bracht (Ed.), *Health promotion at the community level*. Newbury Park, CA: Sage.

Antonovsky, A. (1976). *Health, Stress, and Coping*. San Francisco: Jossey Bass.

Ashby, W. R. (1958). General systems theory as a new discipline. *General Systems, 3,* 1-6.

Ashton, J. (Ed.). (1992). *Healthy cities*. Philadephia, PA: Open University Press.

ASSIST program guidelines for tobacco-free communities. (1991). Rockville, MD: Prospect.

ASSIST Working Group on Durability. (1996). *Turning point for tobacco control: Toward a national strategy to prevent and control tobacco use*. Rockville, MN: Prospect Associates.

Atwood, K., Colditz, G. A., & Kawachi, I. (1997). From public health science to prevention policy: Placing science in its social and political contexts. *American Journal of Public Health, 87,* 1603-1605.

Bahr, J., & Wehrhahn, R. (1993). Life expectancy and infant mortality in Latin America. *Social Science & Medicine, 36*(10), 1373-1382.

Bandura, A. (1969). *Principles of behavior modification*. New York: Holt.

Bandura, A. (1977). *Social learning theory*. Englewood Cliffs, NJ: Prentice Hall.

Bandura, A. (1986). *Social foundations of thought and action: A social cognitive theory*. Englewood Cliffs, NJ: Prentice Hall.

Bandura, A. (1992). A social cognitive approach to the exercise of control over AIDS infection. In R. J. DiClemente (Ed.), *Adolescents and AIDS: A generation in jeopardy* (pp. 89-116). Newbury Park, CA: Sage.

Bandura, A. (1994). Social cognitive theory of mass communication. In J. Bryant & D. Zillman (Eds.), *Media effects: Advances in theory and research* (pp. 61-90). Hillsdale, NJ: Lawrence Erlbaum.

Barnett, T., & Blaikie, P. (1992). *AIDS in Africa: Its present and future impact*. London: Belhaven.

Barsky, A. J. (1988). *Worried sick: Our quest for wellness*. Boston: Little, Brown.

Basch, C. E., Sliepcevich, E. M., Gold, R. S., Duncan, D. F., & Kolbe, L. J. (1985). Avoiding type III errors in health education program evaluation: A case study. *Health Education Quarterly, 12,* 315-331.

Basch, P. F. (1991). A historical perspective on international health. *Infectious Disease Clinics of North America, 5*(2), 183-196.

Batten, T. R. (1967). *The non-directive approach in group and community work*. Oxford: Oxford University Press.

Becker, G. S. (1977). *The economic approach to human behavior*. Chicago: University of Chicago Press.

Becker, M. H. (1974). *The health belief model and personal health behavior*. Thorofare, NJ: Slack.

Belizan, J. M., Barros, F., Langer, A., Farnot, U., Victoria, C., & Villar, J. (1995). Obstetrics impact of health education during pregnancy on behavior and utilization of health resources. *American Journal of Obstetrics and Gynecology, 173*(3), 894-899.

Bell, C., & Newby, H. (1971). *Community studies: An introduction to the sociology of the local community*. New York: Praeger.

Bennett, F. J. (Ed.). (1979). *Community diagnosis and health action: A manual for tropical and rural areas*. London: McMillan.

Beresford, S. A., Curry, S. J., Kristal, A. R., Lazovich, D., Feng, Z., & Wagner, E. H. (1997). A dietary intervention in primary care practice: The Eating Patterns Study. *American Journal of Public Health, 87,* 610-616.

Bergsjø, P. (1996). *Action against AIDS: The MUTAN report*. Bergen: University of Bergen, Center for International Health.

Bergsjø, P., Olomi, R.M.S., Talle, A., & Klepp, K.-I. (1995). Bar workers as health educators: Prevention of sexually transmitted diseases in high-risk areas. *Tanzanian Medical Journal, 10,* 14-18.

Bettencourt, B. A. (1996). Grassroots organizations: Recurrent themes and research approaches. *Journal of Social Issues, 52*(1), 207-220.

Biddle, W. W., & Biddle, L. (1985). *The community development process: the rediscovery of local initiative*. New York: Holt, Rhinehart & Winston.

Bjarveit, K. (1986). Effect of intervention on coronary heart disease risk factors in some Norwegian counties. *American Journal of Medicine, 80,* 12-17.

Bjärås, G. (1991). The need for leadership for motivation of participants in a community intervention programme. *Scandinavian Journal for Social Medicine, 19*, 190-198.

Blackburn, H. (1983). Research and demonstration projects in community cardiovascular disease prevention. *Journal of Public Health Policy, 4*, 398-421.

Blackburn, H. (1992). Community programs in coronary heart disease prevention and health promotion: Changing community behavior. In M. G. Marmot & P. Elliot (Eds.), *Coronary heart disease epidemiology: From aetiology to public health* (pp. 495-514). Oxford: Oxford University Press.

Blackburn, H., Luepker, R., Kline, F. G., Bracht, N., Carlaw, R., Jacobs, D., Mittelmark, M., Stauffer, L., & Taylor, H. L. (1984). The Minnesota Heart Health Program: A research and demonstration project in cardiovascular disease prevention. In J. D. Matarazzo, S. M. Weiss, A. J. Herd, N. Mier, & S. M. Weiss (Eds.), *Behavioral health: A handbook for health enhancement and disease prevention.* Silver Spring, MD; John Wiley.

Blaine, T. M., Forster, J. L., Hennrikus, D., O'Neil, S., Wolfson, M., & Pham, H. (1997). Creating tobacco control policy at the local level: Implementation of a direct action organizing approach. *Health Education & Behavior, 24*(5), 640-651.

Blum, H. L. (1981). Planning as a preferred instrument for achieving social change. In H. L. Blum (Ed.), *Planning for health: Generics for the eighties* (pp. 39-85). New York: Human Sciences.

Blystad, A. (1995). Peril or penalty: AIDS in the context of social change among the Barabaig. In K.-I. Klepp, P. M. Biswalo, & A. Talle (Eds.), *Young people at risk: Fighting AIDS in Northern Tanzania* (pp. 86-106). Oslo: Scandinavian University Press.

Boonstra, E. (1990). *The development of a community diagnosis as a tool in health planning in Askvoll municipality* (M.P.H. thesis; in Norwegian). Nordic School of Public Health, Gothenburg, Sweden.

Bossert, T. J. (1990). Can they get along without us? Sustainability of donor-supported health projects in Central America and Africa. *Social Science Medicine, 30*, 1015-1023.

Bossert, T. J., Hsiao, W., Barrera, M., Alarcon, L., Casares, M. L., & Casares, C. (1998). Transformation of ministries of health in the era of health reform: The case of Colombia. *Health Policy and Planning, 13*(1), 59-77.

Boulding, K. E. (1978). General systems theory: The skeleton of science. In J. Shafritz & P. Whitbeck (Eds.), *Classics of organization theory* (pp. 121-131). Oak Park, IL: Moore.

Bracht, N. (1988). Community analysis precedes community organisation for cardiovascular disease prevention. *Scandinavian Journal of Primary Health Care, Suppl. 1*, 23-30.

Bracht, N. F., Finnegan, J. R., Rissel, C., Weisbrod, R., Gleason, J., Corbett, J., & Veblen-Mortenson, S. (1994). Community ownership and program continuation following a health demonstration program. *Health Education Research, 9*(2), 243-255.

Bracht, N., & Kingsbury, L. (1990). Community organization principles in health promotion: A five-stage model. In N. Bracht (Ed.), *Health promotion at the community level* (pp. 66-90). Newbury Park, CA: Sage.

Bracht, N., Thompson, B., & Winner, C. (1996). *Planning for durability: Keeping the vision alive.* Rockville, MD: Prospect.

Bracht, N., & Tsouros, A. (1990). Principles and strategies of effective community participation. *Health Promotion International, 5*(3), 199-208.

Brown, E. R. (1991). Community action for health promotion: A strategy to empower individuals and communities. *International Journal of Health Services, 21*(3), 441-456.

Bruhn, J. G., & Brandon, J. E. (Eds.). (1997). *Border health: Challenges for the United States and Mexico.* New York: Garland.

Bryan, R. T., Balderrama, F., Tonn, R. J., & Dias, J. C. (1994). Community participation in vector control: Lessons from Chagas' disease. *American Journal of Tropical Medicine & Hygiene, 50*(6 Suppl.), 61-71.

Buasai, S. (1997). An organised approach to setting up a health promotion organisation in Thailand. *Health Promotion Matters, 1*(3), 18-20.

Buller, P. F., & McEvoy, G. M. (1989). Determinants of the institutionalization of planned organizational change. *Group Organizational Studies, 14*, 33-50.

Burdus, A. (1990, October). What can and cannot be achieved by advertising. *Proceedings of the Nutrition Society, 49*(3), 403-9.

Bureau of Statistics (Tanzania). (1990). *Population census: Arusha and Kilimanjaro regional profiles.* Dar es Salaam: President's Office, Planning Commission.

Burt, R. S., & Minor, M. J. (1983). *Applied network analysis: A methodological introduction.* Beverly Hills, CA: Sage.

Butterfoss, F. D., Goodman, R. M., & Wandersman, A. (1993). Community coalitions for prevention and health promotion. *Health Education Research: Theory and Practice, 8*(3), 315-330.

Byrd, T. (1992). Project *Verdad*: A community development approach to health. *Hygiene, 11*(4), 15-20.

Cambre, M. (1981). Historical overview of formative evaluation of instructional media products. *Education Communications and Technology Journal, 29*, 3-25.

Campbell, D., & Stanley, J. C. (1963). *Experimental and quasi-experimental designs for research.* Chicago: Rand McNally.

Campfens, H. (Ed.). (1997). *Community development around the world: Practice, theory, research, training.* Toronto: University of Toronto Press.

Cancian, F. M. (1960). Functional analysis of change. *American Sociological Review, 25*, 818-827.

Cardaci, D. (1994). Health education program with female workers at a Mexican university. *Promotion & Education, 1*(3), 5-9.

Cardaci, D. (1997). Health education in Latin America: The difficulties of community participation and empowerment. *Promotion & Education, 4*(1), 20-22.

Carlaw, R. W., Mittelmark, M. B., Bracht, N., & Luepker, R. (1984). Organization for a community cardiovascular health program: Experiences from the Minnesota Heart Health Program. *Health Education Quarterly, 11*, 243-252.

Carleton, R. A., Lasater, T. M., Assaf, A. R., Feldman, H. A., McKinlay, S., & the Pawtucket Heart Health Program Writing Group. (1995). The Pawtucket Heart Health Program: Community changes in cardiovascular disease risk factors and projected disease risk. *American Journal of Public Health, 85*, 777-785.

Carlyn, M., & Bracht, N. (1995, July). *Coalition pilot assessment project.* Unpublished report for National Cancer Institute re ASSIST Project by Prospect Associates, Rockville, MD.

Carrageta, M. O., Negrao, L., & de-Padua, F. (1994). Community-based stroke prevention: A Portuguese challenge. *Health Reports, 6*(1), 189-195.

Carter, R. F., Stamm, K. R., & Heintz-Knowles, K. (1992, December). Agenda-setting and consequentiality. *Journalism Quarterly, 69*(4), 868-877.

Castiglia, P. T. (1994). Health care on the Mexican-American border. In B. Bullough & C. L. Bullough (Eds.), *Nursing issues for the nineties and beyond* (pp. 199-211). New York: Springer.

Center for Disease Control and Prevention. (1995). *Morbidity and mortality weekly report recommendations and reports, prevention and managed care: Opportunities for managed care organizations, purchasers of health care, and public health agencies.* HHS. Public Health Service, 44: RR-14. Washington, D.C.: Government Printing Office.

Centers for Disease Control. (1992). PATCH: Planned Approach To Community Health. *Journal of Health Education, 23*(3), 129-132.

Central Bureau of Statistics, Norway. (1993). *Social survey, 1993.* Oslo: Statistics Norway.

Cervical cancer control: Status and directions (NIH pub. no. 91-3223). (1991). Bethesda, MD: National Cancer Institute.

Chamberlain, M. A. (1996, January). Health communication: Making the most of new media technologies: An international overview. *Journal of Health Communication, 1*(1), 43-50.

Chavis, D. M., & Wandersman, A. (1990). Sense of community in the urban environment: A catalyst for participation and community development. *American Journal of Community Psychology, 18*(1), 55-81.

Cheadle, A., Psaty, B., Wagner, E., Diehr, P., Koepsell, T., Curry, S., & Von Korff, M. (1990). Evaluating community-based nutrition programs: Assessing the reliability of a survey of grocery store product displays. *American Journal of Public Health, 80*, 709-711.

Chelala, C. A. (1990). *Adult health in the Americas.* Washington, DC: Pan American Health Organization.

Chen, Z. M., Xu, Z., Collins, R., Li, W. X., & Peto, R. (1997, November 12). Early health effects of the emerging tobacco epidemic in China: A 16-year prospective study. *Journal of the American Medical Association, 278*(18), 1500-1504.

Cheru, F. (1989). The role of the IMF and World Bank in the agrarian crisis of Sudan and Tanzania: Sovereignty vs. control. In B. Onimode (Ed.), *The IMF, the World Bank and the African debt. Vol. 2: The social and political impact* (pp. 77-94). London: Institute for African Alternatives.

Clark, R. A., Geller, B. M., Peluso, N. J., McVety, D. M., & Worden, J. K. (1995). Development of a community mammography registry: Experience in the Breast Screening Program Project. *Radiology, 196*, 811-815.

Clarke, J. N. (1991, August). Media portrayal of disease from the medical, political economy, and life-style perspectives. *Qualitative Health Research, 1*(3), 287-308.

Coelho, P. (1993). *The alchemist*. New York: Harper Collins.

Cohen, A. S., Felix, M.R.J., & Yopp, R. (1986). Measuring community change in disease prevention and health promotion. *Preventive Medicine, 15*, 411-421.

Cohen, R. Y., Stunkard, A., & Felix, M.R.J. (1986). Measuring community change in disease prevention and health promotion. *Preventive Medicine, 15*, 411-421.

Collaboration Work Group of the State Community Health Services Advisory Committee, Minnesota Department of Health. (1996, December). *Developing partnerships to improve public health*. St. Paul, MN: Minnesota Department of Health.

COMMIT Research Group. (1991). Community Intervention Trial for Smoking Cessation (COMMIT): Summary of design and intervention. *Journal of the National Cancer Institute, 83*, 1620-1628.

COMMIT Research Group. (1995). Community Intervention Trial for Smoking Cessation (COMMIT): I. Cohort results from a four-year community intervention. *American Journal of Public Health, 85*, 183-192.

Committee on Performance Measurement. (1996, July). *HEDIS 3.0*. Washington, DC: National Committee on Quality Assurance.

Commonwealth Department of Human Services and Health. (1994). *Better health outcomes for Australians: National goals, targets and strategies for better health outcomes into the next century*. Canberra: Australian Government Publishing Service.

Community Development in Health Project. (1988). *A resource collection*. Melbourne, Australia: Author.

Cook, K. S. (1977). Interorganizational relations. *Sociological Quarterly, 18*, 62-82.

Cook, T. D., & Campbell, D. T. (1979). *Quasi-experimentation: Design and analysis issues for field settings*. Chicago: Rand McNally.

Cottrell, L. S. Jr. (1983). The competent community. In R. Warren & L. Lyons (Eds.), *New perspectives in the American community*. Florence, KY: Dorsey.

Cox, F. M., Erlich, J. L., Rothman, J., & Tropman, J. E. (Eds.). (1979). *Strategies of community organization: a book of readings* (3rd ed.). Itasca, IL: Peacock.

Coye, M. J. (1995). Our own worst enemies: Obstacles to improving the health of the public. In M. J. Coye, W. H. Foege, & W. L. Roper (Eds.), *Leadership in public health*. New York, NY: Milbank Memorial Fund.

Curtice, L. (1993). Strategies and values: research and the WHO Healthy Cities project in Europe. In J. K. Davies & M. P. Kelly (Eds.), *Healthy Cities: Research and practice*. London: Routledge.

Curto de Casas, S. (1993). Geographical inequalities in mortality in Latin America. *Social Science and Medicine, 36*(10), 1349-1355.

Dahrendorf, R. (1959). *Class and class conflict in industrial society*. Stanford, CA: Stanford University Press.

Danigelis, N. L., Roberson, N. L., Worden, J. K., Flynn, B. S., Dorwaldt, A. L., Ashley, J. A., Skelly, J. M., & Mickey, R. M. (1995). Breast screening by African-American women: Insights from a household survey and focus groups. *American Journal of Preventive Medicine, 11*(5), 311-317.

Danigelis, N. L., Worden, J. K., & Mickey, R. M. (1996). The importance of age as a context for understanding African-American women's mammography screening behavior. *American Journal of Preventive Medicine, 12*, 358-366.

Dasher, E. S. (1995). Re-inventing primary care. *Alternative Therapies in Health & Medicine, 1*(5), 29-34.

Dasher, E. S. (1996a). Post modern medicine. *Journal of Alternative & Complementary Medicine, 2*(4), 531-537.

Dasher, E. S. (1996b). *The whole healing system,* http:www.healthy.net/dacher.

Davies, J. K., & Kelly, M. P. (Eds.). (1993). *Healthy Cities: Research and practice.* London: Routledge.

Davis, S. K., Winkleby, M. A., & Farquhar, J. W. (1995, September). Increasing disparity in knowledge of cardiovascular disease risk factors and risk-reduction strategies by socioeconomic status: Implications for policymakers. *American Journal of Preventive Medicine, 11*(5), 318-325.

de la Barra, X. (1998). Poverty: The main cause of ill health in urban children. *Health Education & Behavior, 25,* 46-59.

Department of Health. (1992). *The health of the nation: A strategy for health in England.* London: Her Majesty's Stationery Office.

Dhooper, S., & Tran, T. M. (1998). Understanding and responding to the health and mental helath needs of Asian refugees. *Social Work in Health Care, 27*(4), 65-82.

DiClemente, C. C., & Prochaska, J. O. (1982). Self-change and therapy change of smoking behavior: A comparison of processes of change in cessation and maintenance. *Addictive Behavior, 7,* 133-142.

Dignan, M., & Carr, P. (1986). *Program planning for health education and health promotion.* Philadelphia: Lea & Febiger.

Dluhy, M. J., & Kravitz, S. L. (1990). *Building coalitions in the human services.* Newbury Park, CA: Sage.

Domhoff, W. D. (1969). Where a pluralist goes wrong. *Berkeley Journal of Sociology, 14,* 35-57.

Donohue, G. A., Olien, C. N., & Tichenor, P. J. (1990, May). *Knowledge gaps and smoking behavior.* Paper presented to the annual conference of the American Association for Public Opinion Research (AAPOR), Lancaster, PA.

Draper, R., Curtice, L., Hooper, J., & Goumans, M. (1993). WHO Healthy Cities Project: Review of the first five years (1987-1992). Copenhagen: World Health Organization.

Duhl, L. (1985). Healthy cities. *Health Promotion, 1,* 55-60.

Duhl, L. J. (1996). An ecohistory of health: The role of "Health Cities." *American Journal of Health Promotion, 10*(4), 258-261.

Durch, J. S., Bailey, L. A., & Stoto, M. A. (Eds.). (1997). *Improving health in the community: A role for performance monitoring.* Washington, DC: National Academy Press.

Dwyer, T., Pierce, J. P., Hannam, C. D., & Burke, N. (1986). Evaluation of the Sydney "Quit. for Life" anti-smoking campaign. Part 2. Changes in smoking prevalence. *Medical Journal of Australia, 144,* 344-347.

Ebrahim, S. (1998). Alcohol consumption by pregnant women in the U.S. during 1988-1995. *Obstetrics and Gynecology, 92*(2), 187-192.

Echeverria-Cota. (1996). *Regional brief: Latin America and the Caribbean.* Washington, DC: World Bank.

Egger, G., Fitzgerald, W., Frape, G., Monaem, A., Rubinstein, P., Tyler, C., & McKay, B. (1983). Results of large scale media antismoking campaign in Australia: North Coast "Quit for Life" programme. *British Medical Journal, 287,* 1125-1128.

Ekman, R. (1996). *Injuries in Skaraborg county, Sweden* (thesis). Sundbyberg, Sweden: Karolinska Institutet, Department of Public Health Sciences.

Elder, J. P., McGraw, S. A., Abrams, D. B., Ferreira, A., Lasater, T. M., Longpre, H., Peterson, G. S., Schwertfeger, R., & Carleton, R. A. (1986). Organizational and community approaches to community-wide prevention of heart disease: The first two years of the Pawtucket Heart Health Program. *Preventive Medicine, 15,* 107-117.

Elder, J. P., Schmid, T. L., Dower, P., & Hedlund, S. (1993). Community heart health programs: Components, rationale, and strategies for effective interventions. *Journal of Public Health Policy, 14*(4), 463-479.

Emery, E., & Emery, M. (1996). *The press in America* (8th ed.). Boston: Allyn & Bacon.

Eng, E., & Parker, E. (1994). Measuring community competence in the Mississippi Delta: The interface between program evaluation and empowerment. *Health Education Quarterly, 21*(2), 199-220.

Eng, E., Salmon, M. E., & Mullan, F. (1992). Community empowerment: The critical base for primary health care. *Family and Community Health, 15*(1), 1-12.

Engebretson, J. (1994). Folk healing and biomedicine: Culture clash or complementary approach? *Journal of Holistic Nursing, 12*(3), 240-250.

Engebretson, J. (1997). A multiparadigm approach to nursing. *Advances in Nursing Science, 20*(1), 21-33.

Epp, J. (1986). Achieving health for all: A framework for health promotion. *Scandinavian Journal of Public Health, 77*, 393-407.

Epstein, F. H. (1992). Contribution of epidemiology to understanding coronary heart disease. In M. Marmot & P. Elliott (Eds.), *Coronary heart disease epidemiology* (pp. 20-32). Oxford: Oxford University Press.

Ermann, M. D., & Lundman, R. J. (Eds.). (1978). *Corporate and governmental deviance: Problems of organizational behavior in contemporary society.* New York: Oxford University Press.

Eskenazi, B., Guendelman, S., & Elkin, E. P. (1993). A preliminary study of reproductive outcomes of female maquiladora workers in Tijuana, Mexico. *American Journal of Industrial Medicine, 24*(6), 667-676.

Fahlberg, L. L., Poulin, A. L., Girdano, D. A., & Dusek, D. E. (1991). Empowerment as an emerging approach in health education. *Journal of Health Education, 22*(3), 185-193.

Farquhar, J. W. (1978). The community-based model of lifestyle intervention trials. *American Journal of Epidemiology, 108*, 103-111.

Farquhar, J., Flora, J., & Good, L. (1985). *Integrated comprehensive health promotion programs* (monograph). Palo Alto, CA: Kaiser Family Foundation.

Farquhar, J. W., Fortmann, S. P., Maccoby, N., Haskell, W. L., Williams, P. T., Flora, J. A., Taylor, C. B., Brown, B. W., Solomon, D. S., & Hulley, S. B. (1985). The Stanford Five-City Project: Design and methods. *American Journal of Epidemiology, 122*, 323-334.

Farquhar, J. W., Maccoby, N., & Wood, P. D. (1985). Education and communication studies. In W. W. Holland, R. Detels, & G. Knox (Eds.), *Oxford textbook of public health* (Vol. 3, pp. 207-221). Oxford: Oxford University Press.

Farquhar, J. W., Maccoby, N., Wood, P. D., Alexander, J. K., Breitrose, H., Brown, B. W. Jr., Haskell, W. L., McAlister, A. L., Meyer, A. J., Nash, J. D., & Stern, M. P. (1977). Community education for cardiovascular health. *Lancet, 1*, 1192-1195.

Farquhar, J. W., Wood, P. D., Breitrose, H., Haskell, W. L., Meyer, A. J., Maccoby, N., Alexander, J. K., Brown, B. W., McAlister, A. L., Nash, J. D., & Stem, M. P. (1977). Community education for cardiovascular health. *Lancet, 1*, 1192-1195.

Fawcett, S. B., Francisco, V. T., Paine-Andrews, A., Lewis, R. K., Richter, K. P., Harris, K. J., Williams, E. L., Berkley, J. Y., Schultz, J. A., Fisher, J. L., & Lopez, C. M. (1995). *Work group evaluation handbook: Evaluating and supporting community initiatives for health and development.* Lawrence, KS: Work Group on Health Promotion & Community Development, University of Kansas.

Fawcett, S. B., Lewis, R. K., Paine-Andrews, A., Francisco, V. T., Richter, K. P., Williams, E. L., & Copple, J. (1997). Evaluating community coalitions for the prevention of substance abuse: The case of Project Freedom. *Health Education and Behavior, 24*, 812-828.

Fawcett, S. B., Paine-Andrews, A., Francisco, V. T., Schultz, J. A., Richter, K. P., Lewis, R. K., Williams, E. L., Harris, K. J., Berkley, J. Y., Fisher, J. L., & Lopez, C. M. (1995). Using empowerment theory in collaborative partnerships for community health and development. *American Journal of Community Psychology, 23*, 677-697.

Fawcett, S. B., Paine-Andrews, A., Francisco, V. T., Schultz, J. A., Richter, K. P., Lewis, R. K., Harris, K. J., Williams, E. L., Berkley, J. Y., Lopez, C. M., & Fisher, J. L. (1996). Empowering community health initiatives through evaluation. In E. M. Fetterman, S. J. Kafterian, & A. Wandersman (Eds.), *Empowerment evaluation: Knowledge and tools for self-assessment & accountability* (pp. 161-187). Thousand Oaks, CA: Sage.

Feighery, E., Rogers, T., Thompson, B., & Bracht, N. (1992). *Coalition problem solving guide.* Stanford, CA: Health Promotion Resource Center, Stanford University.

Ferreira-Pinto, J. B., & Ramos, R. (1995). HIV/AIDS prevention among female sexual partners of injection drug users in Ciudad Juarez. *AIDS Care, 7*(4), 477-488.

Finnegan, J. R., Bracht, N., & Viswanath, K. (1989). Community power and leadership analysis in lifestyle campaigns. In C. T. Salmon (Ed.), *Information campaigns: Balancing social values and social change.* Newbury Park, CA: Sage.

Finnegan, J. R., Murray, D. M., Kurth, C., & McCarthy, P. (1989). Measuring and tracking education program implementation: the Minnesota Heart Health Program experience. *Health Education Quarterly, 16*, 77-90.

Finnegan, J. R., Viswanath, K., Kahn, E., & Hannan, P. (1993). Exposure to sources of heart disease prevention information: Community type and social group differences. *Journalism Quarterly, 70*(3), 569-584.

Fishbein, M. (1990). AIDS and behavior change: An analysis based on the theory of reasoned action. *Interamerican Journal of Psychology, 24*, 37-56.

Fishbein, M., & Middlestadt, S. E. (1989). Using the Theory of Reasoned Action as a framework for understanding and changing AIDS-related behaviors. In V. M. Mays, G. W. Albee, & S. F. Schneider (Eds.), *Primary prevention of AIDS: Psychological approaches* (pp. 93-110). Newbury Park, CA: Sage.

Fisher, E. B., Strunk, R. C., Sussman, L. K., Arfken, C., Sykes, R. K., Munro, J. M., Haywood, S., Harrison, D., & Bascom, S. (1996). Acceptability and feasibility of a community approach to asthma management: The neighborhood Asthma Coalition (NAC). *Journal of Asthma, 33*(6), 367-383.

Flora, J. A., Lefebvre, R. C., Murray, D. M., Stone, E. J., Assaf, A., Mittelmark, M. B., & Finnegan, J. R. (1993). A community education monitoring system: methods from the Stanford Five-City Project, the Minnesota Heart Health Program, and the Pawtucket Heart Health Program. *Health Education Research, 8*, 81-95.

Florin, P., & Wandersman, A. (1990). An introduction to citizen participation, voluntary organizations, and community development: Insights for empowerment through research. *American Journal of Community Psychology, 18*(1), 41-53.

Flynn, B. C. (1993). Healthy Cities within the American context. In J. K. Davies & M. P. Kelly (Eds.), *Healthy Cities: Research and practice.* London: Routledge.

Flynn, B. C. (1996). Healthy Cities: Toward worldwide health promotion. *Annual Review of Public Health, 17*, 229-309.

Flynn, B. C., Ray, D. W., & Rider, M. S. (1994). Empowering communities—Action research through healthy cities. *Health Education Quarterly, 21*, 395-405.

Flynn, B. C., Rider, M., & Ray, D. W. (1991). Healthy Cities: The Indiana model of community development in public health. *Health Education Quarterly, 18*, 331-347.

Flynn, B. S., Gavin, P., Worden, J. K., Ashikaga, T., Gautam, S., & Carpenter, J. (1997). Community education programs to promote mammography participation in rural New York State. *Preventive Medicine, 26*, 102-108.

Forster, J. L., Murray, D. M., Wolfson, M., Blaine, T. M., Wagenaar, A. C., & Hennrikus, D. J. (in press). Effects of community policies to reduce youth access to tobacco. *American Journal of Public Health.*

Forsyth, M. C., Fulton, D. L., Lane, D. S., Burg, M. A., & Krishna, M. (1992). Changes in knowledge, attitudes and behavior of women participating in a community outreach education program on breast cancer screening. *Patient Education and Counseling, 19*, 241-250.

Fortmann, S. P., Flora, J. A., Winkleby, M. A., Schooler, C., Taylor, C. B., & Farquhar, J. W. (1995). Community intervention trials: Reflections on the Stanford Five-City experience. *American Journal of Epidemiology, 142*, 576-586.

Fortmann, S. P., Taylor, C. B., Flora, J. A., & Jatulis, D. E. (1993). Changes in adult cigarette smoking prevalence after 5 years of community health education: The Stanford Five-City Project. *American Journal of Epidemiology, 137*, 82-96.

Frank, A. G. (1967). Sociology of development. *Catalyst, 3*, 28-42.

Freire, P. (1970/1993). *Pedagogy of the oppressed.* New York: Seabury.

Friere, P. (1973/1994). *Education for critical consciousness.* New York: Seabury.

Freire, P. (1998). *Teachers as cultural workers: Letters to those who dare teach.* Boulder, CO: Westview.

Fuenzalida-Puelma, H., Linares Parada, A. M., & La Vertu, D. S. (1992). Legal norms regarding AIDS in Latin America and the Caribbean. In H. Fuenzalida-Puelma, A. M. Linares Parada, & D. S. La Vertu (Eds.), *Ethics and law in the study of AIDS* (Scientific Pub. No. 530, pp. 23-126). Washington, DC: Pan American Health Organization.

Gail, M. H., Byar, D. P., Pechacek, T. F., & Corle, D. K. (1992). Aspects of statistical design for the Community Intervention Trial for Smoking Cessation (COMMIT). *Controlled Clinical Trials, 13*, 6-21.

Galaskiewicz, J. (1979). *Exchange networks and community politics.* Beverly Hills, CA: Sage.

Galbally, R. (1997). *A firm foundation for health promotion: An organisational approach.* Melbourne: VicHealth.

Gardner, S. E., Green, P. F., & Marcus, C. (Eds.). (1994). *Signs of effectiveness II: Preventing alcohol, tobacco, and other drug use: A risk factor/resiliency-based approach.* Rockville, MD: Center for Substance Abuse Prevention.

Geis, G. (1978). White collar crime: The heavy electrical equipment antitrust cases of 1961. In M. D. Ermann & R. J. Lundman (Eds.), *Corporate and governmental deviance: Problems of organizational behavior in contemporary society.* New York: Oxford University Press.

Gemson, D. H., Elinson, J., & Messeri, P. (1988). Differences in physician prevention practice patterns for white and minority patients. *Journal of Community Health, 13,* 53-64.

Gibson, C. H. (1991). A concept analysis of empowerment. *Journal of Advanced Nursing, 16,* 354-361.

Gillies, P. (1998). Effectiveness of alliances and partnerships for health promotion. *Health Promotion International, 13*(2), 99-120.

Glanz, K., Lewis, F. M., & Rimer, B. K. (Eds.). (1997). *Health behavior and health education: Theory, research and practice* (2nd ed.). San Francisco: Jossey-Bass.

Glanz, K., & Rimer, B. K. (1995, July). *Theory at a glance: A guide for health promotion practice* (NIH pub. no. 95-3896). Washington, DC: U.S. Department of Health and Human Services, Public Health Service, National Institutes of Health.

Glasgow, R. E., Sorensen, G., Giffen, C., Shipley, R. H., Corbett, K., & Lynn, W. (1996). Promoting worksite smoking control policies and actions: The Community Intervention Trial for Smoking Cessation (COMMIT) experience. *Preventive Medicine, 25,* 186-194.

Goodman, R. M., Burdine, J., Meehan, E., & McLeroy, K. R. (1993). Coalitions. *Health Education Research, 8,* 313-314.

Goodman, R. M., McLeroy, K. R., Steckler, A. M., & Hoyle, R. (1993). Development of level of institutionalization scales for health promotion programs. *Health Education Quarterly, 20,* 161-178.

Goodman, R. M., & Steckler, A. M. (1987). A model for the institutionalization of health promotion programs. *Family and Community Health, 11,* 63-78.

Goodman, R. M., & Steckler, A. M. (1988-1989). The life and death of a health promotion program: An institutionalization perspective. *International Quarterly of Health Education, 8,* 5-19.

Goodman, R. M., & Steckler, A. M. (1990). Mobilizing communities for health enhancement: Theories of organizational change. In K. Glanz, F. M. Lewis, & B. K. Rimer (Eds.), *Health behavior and health education: Theory, research, and practice* (pp. 314-341). San Francisco, CA: Jossey-Bass.

Goodman, R. M., Tenney, M., Smith, D. W., & Steckler, A. (1992). The adoption process for health curriculum innovations in schools: A case study. *Journal of Health Education, 23,* 215-220.

Gordon, A. J., Rojas, Z., & Tidwell, M. (1990). Cultural factors in *Aedes Aegypti* and dengue control in Latin America: A case study from the Dominican Republic. *International Quarterly of Community Health Education, 10*(3),193-211.

Gordon, J. E. (1978). *Structures, or why things don't fall down.* New York: Plenum.

Gottlieb, B. H. (1985). Social networks and social support: An overview of research, practice, and policy implications. *Health Education Quarterly, 12,* 5-22.

Goumans, M., & Springett, J. (1997). From projects to policy: "Healthy Cities" as a mechanism for policy change for health? *Health Promotion International, 1284,* 311-322.

Govindaraj, R., Chellaraj, G., & Murray, C. J. (1997). Health expenditures in Latin America and the Caribbean. *Social Science & Medicine, 44*(2), 157-169.

Green, L. W. (1986). The theory of participation: A qualitative analysis of its expression in national and international health politics. *Advances in Health Education and Promotion, 1,* 211-236.

Green, L. (1990). Contemporary developments in health promotion: Definitions and challenges. In N. Bracht (Ed.), *Health promotion at the community level* (pp. 29-44). Newbury Park, CA: Sage.

Green, L. W., George, M. A., Daniel, M., Frankish, C. J., Herbert, C. J., Bowie, W. R., & O'Neill, M. (1995). *Study of participatory research in health promotion.* Vancouver: Royal Society of Canada.

Green, L. W., & Kreuter, M. W. (1991). *Health promotion planning: An educational and environmental approach* (2nd ed.). Mountain View, CA: Mayfield.

Green, L. W., Kreuter, M. W., Deeds, S. G., & Partridge, K. B. (1980). *Health education planning: A diagnostic approach*. Mountain View: Mayfield.

Green, L. W., & McAlister, A. L. (1984). Macro-intervention to support health behavior change: Some theoretical perspectives and practical reflections. *Health Education Quarterly, 11*, 322-339.

Green, S. B., Corle, D. K., Gail, M. H., Mark, S. D., Pee, D., Freedman, L. S., Graubard, B. I., & Lynn, W. R. (1995). Interplay between design and analysis for behavioral intervention trials with community as the unit of randomization. *American Journal of Epidemiology, 142*, 587-593.

Gregorio, D. I., Kegeles, S., Parker, C., & Benn, S. (1990). Encouraging screening mammograms: Results of the 1988 Connecticut breast cancer detection awareness campaign. *Connecticut Medicine, 43*, 370-373.

Gresham, L. S., Molgaard, C. A., Elder, J. P., & Robin, H. S. (1988). Breast cancer and mammography: Summary of the educational impact of a low-cost mammography program. *Health Education, 15*, 32-35.

Grusky, O., & Miller, G. A. (Eds.). (1981). *The sociology of organizations: Basic studies* (2nd ed.). New York: Free Press.

Gusfield, J. R. (1962). Mass society and extremist politics. *American Sociological Review, 27*, 19-30.

Gutierrez, G., Tapia-Conyer, R., Guiscafre, H., Reyes, H., Martinez, H., & Kumate, J. (1996). Impact of oral rehydration and selected public health interventions on reduction of mortality from childhood diarrhoeal diseases in Mexico. *Bulletin of the World Health Organization, 74*(2), 189-197.

Gutzwiller, F., Nater, B., & Martin, J. (1985). Community-based primary prevention of cardiovascular disease in Switzerland: Methods and results of the National Research Program (NRP 1A). *Preventive Medicine, 14*, 482-491.

Haglund, B. (1988). The community diagnosis concept: A theoretical framework for prevention in the health sector. *Scandinavian Journal of Primary Health, 6*(Suppl. 1), 11-21.

Han, S. T., & Erben, R. (1993). Health promotion in the Western Pacific region of WHO: A programme outline. *Promotion Education, Special No.*, 36-41.

Hancock, L., Sanson-Fisher, R., Redman, S., Burton, R., Burton, L., Butler, J., Gibberd, R., Girgis, A., Hensley, M., McClintock, A., Reid, A., Schofield, M., Tripodi, T., & Walsh, R. (1996). Community action for cancer prevention: Overview of the cancer action in rural towns (CART) project, Australia. *Health Promotion International, 11*(4), 277-290.

Hancock, T. (1993). The Healthy City from concept to application: Implications for research. In J. K. Davies & M. P. Kelly (Eds.), *Healthy Cities: Research and practice*. London: Routledge.

Hanna, M. G., & Robinson, B. (1994). *Strategies for community empowerment*. Lewiston, NY: Edwin Mellen.

Haram, L. (1995). Negotiating sexuality in times of economic want: The young and modern Meru women. In K.-I. Klepp, P. M. Biswalo, & A. Talle (Eds.), *Young people at risk: Fighting AIDS in Northern Tanzania* (pp. 31-48). Oslo: Scandinavian University Press.

Harper, C. L. (1989). *Exploring social change*. Englewood Cliffs, NJ: Prentice Hall.

Harris, J. R., Isham, G. J., & Smith, M. (1998, April). Prevention in managed care: Joining forces for value and quality. *American Journal of Preventive Medicine, 14*(Suppl. 3), 22-97.

Harris, E., & Wills, J. (1997). Developing healthy local communities at local government level: Lessons from the past decade. *Australian and New Zealand Journal of Public Health, 21*, 403-412.

Hawe, P., Degeling, D., & Hall, J. (1990) *Evaluating health promotion: a health worker's guide*. Sydney: Maclennan and Petty.

Hawe, P., Noort, M., King, L., & Jordens, C. (1997). Multiplying health gains: The critical role of capacity-building within health promotion programs. *Health Policy, 39*, 29-42.

Heaney, C. A., & Israel, B. A. (1997). Social networks and social support. In K. Glanz, F. M. Lewis, & B. K. Rimer (Eds.), *Health behavior and health education: Theory, research and practice* (2nd ed., pp. 179-205). San Francisco: Jossey-Bass.

Heath, A. (1976). *Rational choice and social exchange*. Cambridge: Cambridge University Press.

Heath, G. W., Wilson, R. H., Smith, J., & Leonard, B. E. (1991). Community-based exercise and weight control: Diabetes risk reduction and glycemic control in Zuni Indians. *American Journal of Clinical Nutrition, 53*, 1642S-1646S.

Heguye, E. S. (1995). Young people's perception of sexuality and condom use in Kahe. In K.-I. Klepp, P. M. Biswalo, & A. Talle (Eds.), *Young people at risk: Fighting AIDS in Northern Tanzania* (pp. 107-122). Oslo: Scandinavian University Press.

Helakorpi, S., & Puska, P. (1995). Health behavior changes in North Karelia. In P. Puska, J. Tuomilehto, A. Nissinen, & E. Vartiaianen (Eds.), *The North Karelia Project: 20 year results and experiences* (pp. 331-343). Helsinki: National Public Health Institute.

Heller, K. (1990, Summer). Limitations and barriers to citizen participation. *Community Psychologist, 2*, 11-12.

Hempel, C. G. (1959). The logic of functional analysis. In E. Gross (Ed.), *Symposium on sociological theory.* New York: Harper.

Henderson, M., Thompson, B., & Kristal, A. (1995). Behavioural intervention versus chemoprevention. In M. Hakama, V. Beral, E. Buiatti, J. Faivre, & D. M. Parkin (Eds.), *Chemoprevention in cancer control* (IARC Scientific Pub. No. 136, pp. 123-130). Lyon, France: International Agency for Research on Cancer.

Herbert, C. P. (1996). Community-based research as a tool for empowerment: The Haida Gwaii diabetes project example. *Canadian Journal of Public Health—Revue Canadienne de Santé Publique, 87*, 109-112.

Herman, K. A., Wolfson, M., & Forster, J. L. (1993). The evolution, operation and future of Minnesota SAFPLAN: A coalition for family planning. *Health Education Research: Theory & Practice, 8*(3), 331-344.

Hilgartner, S., & Bosk, C. L. (1988). The rise and fall of social problems: A public arenas model. *American Journal of Sociology, 94*(1), 53-78.

Hillebrand, P. L. (1994). Strategic planning: A road map to the future. *Nursing Management, 25*, 30-32.

Hillery, J. A. (1955). Definitions of community: Areas of agreement. *Rural Sociology, 20*(2), 118-127.

Hoffmeister, H., Mensink, G. B., Stolzenberg, H., Hoeltz, J., Kreuter, H., Laaser, U., Nussel, E., Hullemann, K. D., & Troschke, J. V. (1996). Reduction of coronary heart disease risk factors in the German cardiovascular disease prevention study. *Preventive Medicine, 25*, 135-145.

Hofstede, G. (1993). Cultural constraints in management theories. *The Executive, 7*(1), 81-94.

Holm, L.-E. (1991). Community-based cancer prevention: The Stockholm Cancer Prevention Project. *Cancer Detection and Prevention, 15*, 455-457.

Holm, L.-E., Callmer, E., Eriksson, C.-G., Haglund, B. J., Kanstrom, L., & Tillgren, P. (1989). Community-based strategies for cancer prevention in an urban area: The Stockholm Cancer Prevention Program. *Journal of the National Cancer Institute, 81*, 103-106.

House, J. S., Umberson, D., & Landis, K. R. (1988). Structures and processes of social support. *Annual Review of Sociology, 14*, 293-318.

ISA Associates. (1992). *Second annual report of the national evaluation of the Community Partnership Demonstration Program.* Washington, DC: Center for Substance Abuse and Prevention, U.S. Department of Health and Human Services.

Jackson, C., Fortmann, S. P., Flora, J. A., Melton, R. J., Snider, J. P., & Littlefield, D. (1994). The capacity-building approach to intervention maintenance implemented by the Stanford Five-City Project. *Health Education Research, 9*, 385-396.

Jackson, T., Mitchell, S., & Wright, M. (1989). The community development continuum. *Community Health Studies, 13*(1), 66-73.

Jacobs, D. R., Luepker, R. V., Mittelmark, M. B., Folsom, A. R., Pirie, P. L., Mascioli, S. R., Hannan, P. J., Pechacek, T. F., Bracht, N. F., Carlaw, R. W., Kline, F. G., & Blackburn, H. (1986). Community-wide strategies: Evaluation design of the Minnesota Heart Health Project. *Journal of Chronic Diseases, 39*, 775-788.

Janes, G. R. (1997, Spring/Summer). Public health and managed care: Data sharing for common goals. *Chronic Disease Notes & Reports, 10*(1), 6-8.

Jansson, B. (1994). *Expenditure in the community for personal injuries: A pilot study* (Report No. 9; in Swedish). Stockholm, Sweden: National Institute for Public Health 1994:9.

Janz, N. K., & Becker, M. H. (1984). The health belief model: A decade later. *Health Education Quarterly, 11*(1), 1-47.

Jernigan, D. H., & Wright, P. A. (1996). Media advocacy: Lessons from community experiences. *Journal of Public Health Policy, 17*(3), 306-330.

Jochelson, K. (1991). HIV and syphilis in the Republic of South Africa: The creation of an epidemic. *African Urban Quarterly, 6*(1-2), 20-34.

Kahn, S. (1982). *A guide for grassroots leaders: Organizing.* New York: McGraw-Hill.

Karjalainen, S., & Melkas, T. (1993). Health promotion and prevention in Finland: Inequities in health. In A. Bjørndal (Ed.). *Public health in the Nordic countries* (Report No. U 2/1993). Oslo: National Institute for Public Health.

Kelly, J. G. (1979). T'ain't what you do, it's the way you do it. *American Journal of Community Psychology, 7*, 239-261.

Kerns, V. (1992). Preventing violence against women: A Central American case. In P. A. Counts, J. K. Brown, & T. C. Campbell. (Ed.), *Sanctions and sanctuary.* Boulder: Westview.

Kettner, P., Daley, J. M., & Nichols, A. W. (1985). *Initiating change in organizations and communities: A macro practice model.* Monterey, CA: Brooks/Cole.

Kieffer, C. (1984). Citizen empowerment: A developmental perspective. *Prevention in Human Services, 3*(1), 9-36.

Kinney, G. F., & Gift, R. G. (1997). Building a framework for multiple improvement initiatives. *Joint Commission on Quality Improvement, 23*, 407-423.

Kirkman-Liff, B., & Kronenfeld, J. J. (1992). Access to cancer screening services for women. *American Journal of Public Health, 82*, 733-735.

Kish, L. (1965). *Survey sampling.* New York: Wiley.

Kisil, M., & Chaves, M. (1994). Linking the university with the community and its health system. *Medical Education, 28*(5), 343-349.

Klepp, K., Perry, C. L., & Jacobs, D. R. (1991). Etiology of drinking and driving among adolescents: Implications for primary prevention. *Health Education Quarterly, 18*(4), 415-427.

Klepp, K.-I., Ndeki, S. S., Seha, A. M., Hannan, P., Lyimo, B. A., Msuya, M. H., Irema, M. N., & Schreiner, A. (1994). AIDS education for primary school children in Tanzania: An evaluation study. *AIDS, 8*, 1157-1162.

Klepp, K.-I., Msuya, M. H., Lyimo, B. A., & Bergsjø, P. (1995). AIDS information strategies: Experiences from Arusha and Kilimanjaro. *Tanzanian Medical Journal, 10*, 8-11.

Klepp, K.-I., Ndeki, S. S., Thuen, F., Leshabari, M. T., & Seha, A. M. (1996). Predictors of intention to be sexually active among Tanzanian school children. *East African Medical Journal, 73*, 218-224.

Klepp, K.-I., Ndeki, S. S., Leshabari, M. T., Hannan, P., & Lyimo, B. A. (1997). AIDS education in Tanzania: Promoting risk reduction among primary school children. *American Journal of Public Health, 87*, 1931-1936.

Klouman, E., Masenga, E. J., Klepp, K.-I., Sam, N. E., Nkya, W., & Nkya, C. (1997). HIV and reproductive tract infections in a total village population in rural Kilimanjaro, Tanzania: Women at increased risk. *Journal of Acquired Immune Deficiency Syndromes and Human Retrovirology, 14*, 163-168.

Klouman, E., Masenga, E. J., Sam, N. E., & Lauwo, Z. (1995). Control of sexually transmitted diseases: Experiences from a rural and an urban community. In K.-I. Klepp, P. M. Biswalo, & A. Talle (Eds.), *Young people at risk: Fighting AIDS in Northern Tanzania* (pp. 204-221). Oslo: Scandinavian University Press.

Koepsell, T. D., Diehr, P. H., Cheadle, A., & Kristal, A. (1995). Invited commentary: Symposium of community intervention trials. *American Journal of Epidemiology, 142*, 594-599.

Koepsell, T. D., Martin, D. C., Diehr, P. H., Psaty, B. M., Wagner, E. H., Perrin, E. B., & Cheadle, A. (1991). Data analysis and sample size issues in evaluations of community-based health promotion and disease prevention programs: A mixed-model analysis of variance approach. *Journal of Clinical Epidemiology, 44*(7), 701-713.

Community-wide prevention of cardiovascular disease: education strategies of the Minnesota Heart Health Program. *Preventive Medicine, 15*, 1-17.

Mnyika, K. S., Klepp, K.-I., Kvåle, G., Nilssen, S., Kissila, P., & Ole-Kingóri, N. (1994). Prevalence of HIV-1 infection in urban, semi-urban and rural areas in Arusha region, Tanzania. *AIDS, 8*, 1477-1481.

Mnyika, K. S., Klepp, K.-I., Kvåle, G., Schreiner, A., & Seha, A. M. (1995). Condom awareness and use in the Arusha and Kilimanjaro regions, Tanzania: A population-based study. *AIDS Education and Prevention, 7*, 403-414.

Mnyika, K. S., Klepp, K.-I., Ole-Kingóri, N., & Seha, A. M. (1995). Securing a safe blood supply: Screening of blood donors. In K.-I. Klepp, P. M. Biswalo, & A. Talle (Eds.), *Young people at risk: Fighting AIDS in Northern Tanzania* (pp. 123-132). Oslo: Scandinavian University Press.

Mollel, O. L., Olomi, R.M.S., Mwanga, J. J., & Mongi, B. F. (1995). Peer education in Mererani mining settlement. In K.-I. Klepp, P. M. Biswalo, & A. Talle (Eds.), *Young people at risk: Fighting AIDS in Northern Tanzania* (pp. 196-203). Oslo: Scandinavian University Press.

Montaño, D. E., & Taplin, S. H. (1991). A test of an expanded theory of reasoned action to predict mammography participation. *Social Science and Medicine, 32*, 733-741.

Montaño, D. E., Thompson, B., Taylor, V., & Mahloch, J. (1997). Understanding mammography intention and utilization among women in an inner city public health hospital clinic. *Preventive Medicine, 26*, 817-824.

Moore, W. E. (1963). *Social change.* Englewood Cliffs, NJ: Prentice Hall.

Morris, J. N. (1975). *Uses of epidemiology* (3rd ed.). Edinburgh: Churchill Livingstone.

Morris, L. (1992). Sexual experience use of contraception among young adults in Latin America. *Morbidity and Mortality Weekly Report: CDC Surveillance Summaries, 41*(4), 27-40.

Moure-Eraso, R., Wilcox, M., Punnett, L., Copeland, L., & Levenstein, C. (1994). Back to the future: Sweatshop conditions on the Mexico-U.S. border: Community health impact of maquiladora industrial activity. *American Journal of Industrial Medicine, 25*(3), 311-324.

Mulford, C. L. (1984). *Interorganizational relations: Implications for community development.* New York: Human Sciences.

Murray, C. (Ed). (1997). *The global burden of disease.* New York: Harvard School of Public Health.

Murray, D. M. (1995). Design and analysis of community trials: Lessons from the Minnesota Heart Health Program. *American Journal of Epidemiology, 142*, 569-575.

Murray, D. M., Hannan, P. J., & Baker, W. L. (1996). A Monte Carlo study of alternate responses to intraclass correlation in community trials. *Evaluation Review, 20*(3), 313-337.

Murray, D. M., Hannan, P. J., Jacobs, D. R., McGovern, P. J., Schmid, L., Baker, W. L., & Gray, C. (1994). Assessing intervention effects in the Minnesota Heart Health Program. *American Journal of Epidemiology, 139*, 91-103.

Muto, T., Kikuchi, S., Tomita, M., Fujita, Y., Kurita, M., & Ozawa, K. (1996). Status of health promotion program implementation and future tasks in Japanese companies. *Indonesian Health, 34*(2), 101-111.

Nathan, M. B. (1993). Critical review of *Aedes Aegypti* control programs in the Caribbean and selected neighboring countries. *Journal of the American Mosquito Control Association, 9*(1), 1-7.

Nathan, M. B., & Knudsen, A. B. (1991). *Aedes Aegypti* infestation characteristics in several Caribbean countries and implications for integrated community-based control. *Journal of the American Mosquito Control Association, 7*(3), 400-404.

National AIDS Control Program. (1994). *AIDS surveillance* (Report No. 8). Dar es Salaam: Ministry of Health, Epidemiological Unit NACP.

National AIDS Control Program (NACP) (1997). *HIV/AIDS/STDs Surveillance* (Report No. 11). Dar es Salaam, Tanzania: Ministry of Health, Epidemiological Unit NACP.

National Board of Health, Sweden. (1997). *Public health report 1997* (SoS-report 1997:18). Stockholm: Socialstyrelsen.

National Cancer Institute Breast Cancer Screening Consortium. (1990). Screening mammography: A missed clinical opportunity? *Journal of the American Medical Association, 264*, 54-58.

National Cancer Institute Cancer Screening Consortium for Underserved Women. (1995). Breast and cervical cancer screening among underserved women: Baseline survey results from six states. *Archives of Family Medicine, 4,* 617-624.

National Institute on Alcohol Abuse and Alcoholism. (1994). County alcohol problem indicators, 1986-1990. In *U.S. Alcohol Epidemiological Data Reference Manual* (Vol. 3). Washington, DC: National Institutes of Health, U.S. Department of Health and Human Services, Public Service.

Ndeki, S. S., Klepp, K.-I., & Mliga, G. R. (1994). Knowledge, perceived risk of AIDS and sexual behavior among primary school children in two areas of Tanzania. *Health Education Research, 9,* 133-138.

Ndeki, S. S., Klepp, K.-I., Seha, A. M., & Leshabari, M. T. (1994). Exposure to HIV/AIDS information, AIDS knowledge, perceived risk and attitudes toward people with AIDS among primary school-children in Northern Tanzania. *AIDS Care, 6,* 183-191.

Neilsen, G. A., & Young, F. J. (1994). HIV/AIDS, advocacy and anti-discrimination legislation: The Australian response. *International Journal of STDs and AIDS, 1,* 13-7.

Neuber, K. (1980). *Needs assessment: A model for community planning.* Beverly Hills, CA: Sage.

New South Wales Department of Health. (1986). *Review of area management of health services: Final report* (State Health Pub. No. (PPR) 86-042). Sydney: Government Printing Office.

Ngomuo, E. T., Klepp, K.-I., Rise, J., & Mnyika, K. S. (1995). Promoting safer sexual practices among young adults: A survey of health workers in Moshi rural district, Tanzania. *AIDS Care, 7,* 501-507.

Nilsen, Ø. (1996). Community health promotion: Concepts and lessons from contemporary sociology. *Health Policy, 36,* 167-183.

Nilsen, Ø., & Kraft, P. (1997). Do local inhabitants want to participate in community injury prevention? A focus on the significance of local identities for community participation. *Health Education Research, 12*(3), 333-345.

Nisbet, R. (1973). *The social philosophers.* New York: Crowell.

Nix, H. L. (1978). *The community and its involvement in the study planning action process* (HEW Pub. No. CDC 78-8355). Washington, DC: U.S. Government Printing Office.

Nordic Medico-Statistical Committee (NOMESCO). (1990). *Classification for accident monitoring* (2nd rev.; No. 34., Nord 1990:100). Copenhagen: Author.

Norris, T. (1997). Building healthy cities: A collaborative effort. *The Bulletin, 41*(Suppl. A), 22-23.

Norwegian Ministry of Social Affairs. (1988). *The health policy towards year 2000: National plan for health* (in Norwegian; Report to Parliament No. 41). Oslo: Author.

Norwegian Ministry of Social Affairs. (1993). *Challenges in health promotion and prevention* (in Norwegian; Report to Parliament No. 37). Oslo: Author.

Nutbeam, D., & Wise, M. (1995). Planning for health for all: International experience in setting health goals and targets. In M. Wilkinson (Ed.), *Proceedings of the International Health Promotion Conference: Where social values and personal worth meet.* Brunel.

O'Connell, B. (1978). From service to advocacy to empowerment. *Social Casework, 59*(4), 195-202.

Olson, M. (1965). *The logic of collective action.* Cambridge, MA: Harvard University Press.

O'Neill, M., Pederson, A., & Rootman, I. (1994). Beyond Lalonde: Two decades of Canadian health promotion. In A. Pederson, M. O'Neill, & I. Rootman (Eds.), *Health promotion in Canada: Provincial, national and international perspectives* (pp. 374-386). Toronto: W. B. Sanders.

Östberg, V. (1996). *Social structure and children's life chances: An analysis of child mortality in Sweden.* Stockholm: Department of Sociology, University of Stockholm.

Paalman, M., Bekedam, H., Hawken, L. & Nyheim, D. (1998). A critical review of priority setting in the health sector: The methodology of the 1993 World Development Report. *Health Policy and Planning, 13*(1), 13-31.

Pachter, L. M. (1994). Culture and clinical care: Folk illness beliefs and behaviors and their implications for health care delivery. *Journal of the American Medical Association, 271*(9), 690-694.

Packard, R. M., & Epstein, P. (1991). Epidemiologists, social scientists, and the structure of medical research on AIDS in Africa. *Social Science and Medicine, 33*(7), 771-794.

Paisley, W. J. (1981). Public communication campaigns: The American experience. In R. E. Rice & W. J. Paisley (Eds.), *Public communication campaigns* (pp. 15-40). Beverly Hills, CA: Sage.

Pan American Health Organization. (1991). *Strategic orientations and program priorities, 1991-1994.* Washington, DC: Author.

Pan American Health Organization. (1992). *Health promotion and equity: Declaration of Santafé de Bogotá.* Santafé de Bogotá, Colombia: Ministry of Health of Colombia.

Pan American Health Organization. (1993). *Resolution V: Health of indigenous peoples in the region of the Americas* (Document CD37/20). Washington, DC: Author.

Pan American Health Organization. (1995). *Strategic and programmatic orientations, 1995-1998.* Washington, DC: Author.

Pan American Health Organization. (1997). *Cooperation of the Pan American Health Organization in the health sector reform processes.* Washington, DC: Author.

Parra, P. A. (1993). Midwives in the Mexican health system. *Social Science & Medicine, 37*(11), 1321-1329.

Parsons, T. (1951). *The social system.* New York: Free Press.

Paskett, E. D., Tatum, C. M., Mack, D. W., Hoen, H., Case, L. D., & Velez, R. (1996). Validation of self-reported breast and cervical cancer screening tests among low-income minority women. *Cancer Epidemiology, Biomarkers & Prevention, 5,* 721-726.

Paskett, E. D., McMahon, K., Tatum, C., Velez, R., Shelton, B., Case, L. D., Wofford, J., Moran, W., & Wymer, A. (1998). Clinic-based interventions to promote breast and cervical cancer screening. *Preventive Medicine, 27,* 120-128.

Pellegrini, A., Jr., Goldbaum, M., & Silvi, J. (1997). Production of scientific articles about health in six Latin American countries, 1973-1992 (in Spanish). *Revista Panamericana de Salud Publica, 1*(1), 23-34.

Perkins, D. D., & Zimmerman, M. A. (1995). Empowerment theory, research, and application. *American Journal of Community Psychology, 23*(5), 569-579.

Perry, C. L., & Kelder, S. H. (1992a). Models for effective prevention. *Journal of Adolescent Health, 13,* 355-363.

Perry, C. L., & Kelder, S. H. (1992b). Prevention. In *Annual review of addictions research and treatment* (pp. 453-472). New York: Pergamon.

Perry, C. L., Williams, C. L., Forster, J. L., Wolfson, M., Wagenaar, A. C., Finnegan, J. R., McGovern, P. G., Veblen-Mortenson, S., Komro, K. A., & Anstine, P. (1993). Background, conceptualization, and design of a communitywide research program on adolescent alcohol use: Project Northland. *Health Education Research Theory & Practice, 8*(1), 125-136.

Perry, C. L., Williams, C. L., Veblen-Mortenson, S., Toomey, T., Komro, K. A., Anstine, P. S., McGovern, P. G., Finnegan, J., Forster, J. L., Wagenaar, A. C., & Wolfson, M. (1996). Outcomes of a community-wide alcohol use prevention program during early adolescence: Project Northland. *American Journal of Public Health, 86*(7), 956-965.

Peters, R. (1996). Australia's new gun laws: Preventing the backslide [editorial]. *Australia and New Zealand Public Health, 20*(4), 339-340.

Pick, S., Reyes, J., Alvarez, M., Cohen, S., Craige, J., & Troya, A. (1996). AIDS prevention training for pharmacy workers in Mexico City. *AIDS Care, 8*(1), 55-69.

Pilisuk, M., McCallister, J., & Rothman, J. (1996). Coming together for action: The challenge of contemporary grassroots community organizing. *Journal of Social Issues, 52*(1), 15-37.

Plata, M. I. (1992). Latin American women and AIDS. In H. Fuenzalida-Puelma, A. M. Linares Parada, & D. S. La Vertu (Eds.), *Ethics and law in the study of AIDS* (Scientific Pub. No. 530, pp. 232-235). Washington, DC: Pan American Health Organization.

Ploeg, J., Dobbins, M., Hayward, S., Ciliska, D., Thomas, H., & Underwood, J. (1996). *Effectiveness of community development projects: Systematic overview.* Retrieved July 24, 1998 from the Ontario Health Care Evaluation Network on the World Wide Web, http://hiru.mcmaster.ca/ohcen/groups/hthu/-95-5.htm.

Porras, I. I., & Robertson, P. J. (1987). Organization development theory: A typology and evaluation. In R. W. Woodman & W. A. Pasmore (Eds.), *Research in organizational change and development* (Vol. 1, pp. 146-192). Greenwich, CT: JAI.

Powles, J. W., & Gifford, S. (1993). Health of nations: Lessons from Victoria, Australia. *British Medical Journal, 6870,* 125-127.

Price, C., & Tsouros, A. D. (Eds.). (1996). *Our cities.* Copenhagen: WHO Regional Offices for Europe.

Prochaska, J. O., & DiClemente, C. C. (1983). Stages and process of self-change of smoking: Toward an integrative model of change. *Journal of Consulting and Clinical Psychology, 51,* 390-395.

Prochaska, J. O., DiClemente, C. C., & Norcross, J. C. (1992). In search of how people change: Applications to addictive behaviors. *American Psychologist, 47,* 1102-1114.

Prochaska, J. O., Norcross, J. C., & DiClemente, C. C. (1994). *Changing for good.* New York: Morrow.

Prochaska, J. O., Velicer, W. F., Rossi, J. S., Goldstein, M. G., Marcus, B. H., Rakowski, W., Fiore, C., Harrlow, L. L., Redding, C. A., Rosenbloom, D., & Rossi, S. R. (1994). Stages of change and decisional balance for 12 problem behaviors. *Health Psychology, 13,* 39-46.

Public Health Commission. (1994). *A strategic direction to improve and protect the public health: Policy advice to the Minister of Health, 1993-1994.* Wellington, Australia: Public Health Commission.

Puentes-Markides, C., & Garrett, M. J. (1996). Application of "futures" in the community-level health promotion with special reference to Latin America. *International Journal of Health Planning & Management, 11*(4), 317-338.

Pulido, P. A. (1989). Strategies for developing innovative programs in international medical education: A viewpoint from Latin America. *Academic Medicine, 64*(5 Suppl.), S17-S22.

Puska, P. (Ed.). (1988). Comprehensive cardiovascular community control programmes in Europe (World Health Organization EURO Reports and Studies No. 106). Copenhagen: World Health Organization.

Puska, P. (1995a). General discussion, recommendations, and conclusion. In P. Puska, J. Tuomilehto, A. Nissinen, & E. Vartiaianen (Eds.). *The North Karelia Project: 20 year results and experiences* (pp. 345-356). Helsinki: National Public Health Institute.

Puska, P. (1995b). Main outline of the North Karelia Project. In P. Puska, J. Tuomilehto, A. Nissinen, & E. Vartiaianen (Eds.). *The North Karelia Project: 20 year results and experiences* (pp. 23-30). Helsinki: National Public Health Institute.

Puska, P., Nissinen, A., Tuomilehto, J., Salonen, J. T., Koskela, K., McAlister, A., Kottke, T. E., Maccoby, N., & Farquhar, J. W. (1985). The community-based strategy to prevent coronary heart disease: Conclusions from the ten years of the North Karelia Project. *Annual Review of Public Health, 6,* 147-193.

Puska, P., Salonen, J. T., Nissinen, A., & Tuomilehto, J. (1983). Ten years of the North Karelia Project: Results with community-based prevention of coronary heart disease. *Scandinavian Journal of Social Medicine, 11,* 65-68.

Puska, P., Tuomilehto, J., Salonen, J., Neittaanmaki, L., Maki, J., Virtamo, J., Nissinen, A., Koskel, K.; & Takalo, T. (1979). Changes in coronary risk factors during comprehensive five-year programme to control cardiovascular disease (North Karelia Project). *British Medical Journal, 2,* 1173-1178.

Puska, P., Tuomilehto, J., Salonen, J., Nissinen, A., Virtamo, J., Björkqvist, S., Koskela, K., Neittaanmäki, L., Takalo, L., Kottke, T. E., M ki, J., Sipilä, P., & Varvikko, P. (1981). *The North Karelia Project: Evaluation of a comprehensive community programme for control of cardiovascular diseases in North Karelia, Finland, 1972-1977.* Copenhagen: WHO/EURO.

Puska, P., Toumilehto, J., Nissinen, A., & Vartiainen, E. (Eds.). (1995). *The North Karelia Project: 20 years results and experiences.* Helsinki, Finland: National Public Health Institute (KTL).

Puska, P., Tuomilehto, J., Variainen, E., Korhonen, H. J., & Torppa, J. (1995). Mortality changes. In P. Puska, J. Tuomilehto, A. Nissinen, & E. Vartiaianen (Eds.), *The North Karelia Project: 20 year results and experiences* (pp. 159-167). Helsinki: National Public Health Institute.

Quinn, J. F. (1992). Holding sacred space: The nurse as healing environment. *Holistic Nursing Practice, 6*(4), 26-36.

Quinn, J. F. (1997). Healing: A model for an integrative health care system. *Advanced Practice Nursing Quarterly, 3*(1), 1-7.

Rains, J. W., & Ray, D. W. (1995). Participatory action research for community health promotion. *Public Health Nursing, 12,* 256-261.

Ramirez, A. (1997). *En acción training manual* (NIH Pub. No. 97-4260). Bethesda, MD: National Cancer Institute.

Ramiro Montealegre, J. (1991). Information systems design for development projects in Central America. *Archivos Latinoamericanos de Nutricion, 41*(2), 257-272.

About the Contributors

Chris Borthwick, LL.B., is Manager of the Development Unit of the Victorian Health Promotion Foundation (VicHealth) in Melbourne, Australia. His publications include *Health Promotion for People With Disabilities; The Prevention of Disability; Severe Communication Impairment, Facilitated Communication and Disclosures of Abuse; Re-inventing the Wheelchair,* and "Children in State Institutions: The Mental Health Legislation," in *Disability, Human Rights and Law Reform.*

Janet R. Buelow, Ph.D., M.P.H., M.S.N., R.N., is Associate Professor of Health Services Administration in the School of Business, University of South Dakota, Vermillion. A former fellow of the American Association for the Advancement of Science (AAAS) assigned to the United States Agency for International Development (USAID), she has also engaged in consulting assignments in Latin America, Eastern Europe, Central Asia, and Southeast Asia. Her speciality is aging and long-term care administration. She has published in *Health Marketing Quarterly, Home Health Care Services Quarterly, Journal of Aging and Health, Journal of Applied Gerontology, Journal of Long Term Care Administration,* and *New Directions for Program Evaluation.*

Ralph D'Agostino Jr., Ph.D., is Assistant Professor of Public Health Sciences in the Biostatistics Section at Wake Forest University School of Medicine. His research interests include observational and longitudinal studies and missing data. He is the author or coauthor on more than 45 journal articles, abstracts, and book chapters. He serves as Program Chair for the Epidemiology Section of the American Statistical Association and as an Associate Editor for the *American Journal of Epidemiology.*

Anne L. Dorwaldt, M.A., is a Health Education Coordinator with the Office of Health Promotion Research, University of Vermont, Burlington, Vermont.

John R. Finnegan Jr., Ph.D., is Associate Professor of Epidemiology at the University of Minnesota School of Public Health. He has 18 years of experience in the design, implementation, and evaluation of public health campaigns in the prevention of heart disease, cancer, and youth alcohol use. As a former media professional, he has specialized in the use of mass media in prevention and

271

health promotion. His recent projects have included the Minnesota Heart Health Program, the Cancer and Diet Intervention Project, Project Northland, and the Rapid Early Action for Coronary Treatment (REACT) Study.

Jean Forster, Ph.D., M.P.H., is Associate Professor in the School of Public Health, University of Minnesota. Her research interests center around the potential of public health policy to reduce the population prevalence of chronic disease risk factors. Her recent research has focused on the prevention of tobacco use by youth and the reduction of youth access to tobacco. She is the principal investigator of a National Cancer Institute grant to evaluate the effects of local policy change on youth access to tobacco and adolescent smoking rates and an NCI grant to investigate community strategies to reduce the social availability of tobacco to youth.

Rhonda Galbally, Dip.Ed., D.Sc. Hon, is the founding Chief Executive Officer of the Victorian Health Promotion Foundation (VicHealth) in Melbourne, Australia. She has worked extensively with the World Health Organization to develop guidelines and training. Her work in the health care sector focuses on the integration of health promotion strategies into primary health care programs, development of organizational health capacity at the local level, financing models for health promoiotn, MCH health promotion, and women's health.

Berta M. Geller, Ed.D., is Research Assistant Professor with the Office of Health Promotion Research and the Department of Family Practice and a member of the Vermont Cancer Center, University of Vermont, Burlington, Vermont.

Bo J. A. Haglund, M.D., Ph.D., is Professor in Public Health Sciences and Director of the World Health Organization Collaborating Centre on Supportive Environments at the Karolinska Institute, Sundbyberg, Sweden. He has been a contributor to and editor of several books, including *Community Intervention Strategies* (1986), *Youth Health Promotion: From Theory to Practice in School and Community* (1991), *Work for Health?* (1991), and *Creating Supportive Environments for Health: Stories From the Third International Conference on Health Promotion, Sundsval, Sweden* (1996).

Bridget H.-H. Hsu-Hage, M.S., Ph.D., is the Health Promotion Unit Convener of the Faculty of Medicine, Monash University. She is also the founder and president of the Chinese Health Foundation of Australia. With her medical students, she established the first health promotion home page on the Internet and initiated the *Internet Journal of Health Promotion*. She is a strong advocate for Asian women's health, especially diabetes in pregnancy.

Lee Kingsbury, B.A., is a Community Health Planner in the Division of Community Health Services, Minnesota Department of Health in St. Paul. Her research interests include community organizing, community health planning, and public/private partnerships.

Susan Kinne, Ph.D., is Staff Scientist at the Fred Hutchinson Cancer Research Center in Seattle, Washington.

Knut-Inge Klepp, Ph.D., M.P.H., is Professor in Public Nutrition at the Institute for Nutrition Research, University of Oslo, Norway, and Adjunct Professor in International Health, Center for International Health, University of Bergen, Norway. His research interests center around health promotion among adolescents, reproductive health, and nutrition and food security issues.

Gro Th. Lie, Dr.Psychol., is Associate Professor at the Research Centre for Health Promotion, University of Bergen, Norway. Her current research focus is on HIV prevention and coping strategies for people with AIDS.

Catherine M. Lloyd, M.A., is Assistant Director of the Office of Health Promotion Research at the University of Vermont, Burlington, Vermont.

John G. Maeland, M.D., Ph.D., is Professor in Health Promotion, School of Psychology, University of Bergen, Norway. His research interests include community-oriented health promotion, health and quality of life research, and psychosocial aspects of rehabilitation.

Melkiory C. Masatu, M.D., M.Sc., is with the Center for Educational Development in Health, Arusha, Tanzania. He is currently a Ph.D. student at the University of Bergen, Norway. His research interests include health systems research, with a focus on adolescent use of health care services.

Donna J. Sabina McVety, R.N., Ph.D., was Executive Director of the Lee County Breast Screening Program from December 1990 through June 1997. She is currently serving as volunteer Chairperson of Development for the Lee County Breast Screening Program, Fort Myers, Florida.

Maurice B. Mittelmark, Ph.D., is Professor of Health Promotion, School of Psychology, University of Bergen, Norway. His research interests include community approaches to health promotion and the study of the near social environment's influence on physical and mental health. He is Director of the World Health Organization Collaborating Centre for Health Promotion, University of Bergen. He also directs an international master's degree program in health promotion in which students throughout Europe and Africa participate. His publications include "Realistic outcomes: Lessons From Community-Based Research and Demonstration Programs for the Prevention of Cardiovascular Diseases" (with Hunt, Heath, and Schmid in the *Journal of Public Health Policy,* 1993).

Electra D. Paskett, M.S.P.H., Ph.D., is Associate Professor of Epidemiology and Social Sciences and Health Policy in the Department of Public Health Sicences at Wake Forest University School of Medicine. Her research interests include cancer prevention and screening studies and issues affecting cancer survivors. She is the author or coauthor of more than 46 articles, book chapters, or abstracts. She also serves as the chair of Cancer Control Committee of Cancer and Leukemia Group B.

Cheryl L. Perry, Ph.D., is Professor in the Division of Epidemiology, School of Public Health, at the University of Minnesota. She has published over 125 articles in the peer-reviewed literature on health promotion and prevention programs with children and adolescents, including papers on health promotion and prevention theory, design, implementation, and outcomes. She is principal investigator of the University of Minnesota site of the Child and Adolescent Trial for Cardiovascular Health (CATCH), a 96-school trial to improve eating and exercise patterns of preadolescents; Project HRIDAY-CATCH, a 30-school study in New Delhi, India on cardiovascular health; and Project Northland, a 28-community trial to reduce alcohol use among adolescents.

Phyllis L. Pirie, Ph.D., is Professor in the Division of Epidemiology at the University of Minnesota. She directed the process evaluation of the Minnesota Heart Health Program and has taught evaluation to students in the Community Health Education program at the University of Minnesota School of Public Health for 10 years. She is also Director of the Data Collection and Support Services unit in the Division of Epidemiology, which conducts mail and telephone surveys and carries out data processing operations for research projects in the Division and the Academic Health Center.

Chris Rissel, Ph.D., is an epidemiologist with the Needs Assessment and Health Outcomes Unit of the Central Sydney Area Health Service and Clinical Senior Lecturer with the Department of Public Health and Community Medicine at the University of Sydney. He specializes in research in tobacco control, community participation and empowerment, ethnic health and acculturation, and health outcomes.

Julia Rushing is employed as a biostatistician at the Wake Forest University School of Medicine in the Department of Public Health Sciences. Her collaborations with researchers have led to over 25 coauthored papers in the areas of geriatrics, cancer, diabetes, and cardiovascular disease. She is a member of the American Statistical Association.

Philip W. Setel, Ph.D., is Director of the Adult Morbidity and Mortality Project in Dar es Salaam, Tanzania. His main research focus has been in the area of reproductive health, particularly male sexuality and reproductive rights.

Cathy Tatum, M.A., is Research Associate in the Department of Public Health Sciences at the Wake Forest University School of Medicine. She has worked on several research studies, including the ARIC study, the Polyp Prevention Trial, the Forsyth County Cancer Screening Study, and the Robeson County Outreach, Screening and Education Project. She is author or coauthor of four articles.

Beti Thompson, Ph.D., M.P.H., is Assistant Professor at the University Washington School of Public Health and Community Medicine and an Assistant Member at the Fred Hutchinson Cancer Research Center in Seattle.

Sara Veblen-Mortenson, M.S.W., M.P.H., is the Intervention Director for Project Northland: Partnerships for Community Action and has managed the development and implementation of the intervention components (school, youth, parent, and community) of the research since the beginning of the project in 1990. She has worked with adolescent health issues in school-based clinic and community settings for 10 years.

Ramon Velez, M.D., M.Sc., is Professor of Medicine in the Section of Internal Medicine and Gerontology at the Wake Forest University School of Medicine and Director of Reynolds Health Center. He is author or coauthor of more than 25 articles and abstracts.

K. Viswanath, Ph.D, is Associate Professor in the New School of Communication and the School of Public Health, Ohio State University, Columbus, Ohio.

Abel Arvizu Whittemore, D.B.A., M.H.A., FACHE, is Chair of the Division of Health and Human Services at Walden University, Minneapolis, Minnesota. A former hospital chief executive officer, he has held visiting professorships in Bulgaria and Brazil. He also has served as a Yale/Mellon fellow in international health at Yale University and has engaged in consulting assignments in Latin America, Eastern Europe, Central Asia, and East Africa. His areas of expertise are in health administration and strategic management, and his most recent publication appeared in the *Journal of Long Term Care Administration.*

Carol Winner, M.P.H., is Research Instructor with Georgetown University's National Center for Education in Maternal and Child Health, serving as the Director for the Division of Program and Policy Development. She served as the Director of Technical Assistance on the National Cancer Institute's American Stop Smoking Intervention Study (ASSIST) and has also been a Program Director with the American Lung Association and the Epilepsy Foundation.

Mark Wolfson, Ph.D., is Associate Professor and Director of the Center for Community Research in the Section on Social Sciences and Health Policy, Department of Public Health Sciences, Wake Forest University School of Medicine. His research interests include alcohol and tobacco policy, managed care and population health, and the politics of community health. His recent publications include "Managed Care, Population Health, and Public Health" (in *Research in the Sociology of Health Care*, 1998), "Unintended Consequences and Professional Ethics: Criminalization of Alcohol and Tobacco Use by Youth and Young Adults" (in *Addiction*, 1997), and "Adolescent Smokers' Provision of Tobacco to Other Adolescents" (*American Journal of Public Health*, 1997). His book, *The Fight Against Big Tobacco: The Movement, the State, and the Public's Health* will be published in 1999.

John K. Worden, Ph.D., is Research Professor with the Office of Health Promotion Research and the Department of Family Practice and is a member of the Vermont Cancer Center, University of Vermont, Burlington, Vermont.